woman's contemporary image

Contemporary Programs, Inc.

JEAN ADAMS
MAXINE BREED
DORIE DAMUTH
LOU DAVIS
EVA FARLEY
SIDNEY FAUST
MAGGIE McDONALD, *Senior Editor*
CHARLES A. SAUNDERS

Prentice-Hall, Inc., Englewood Cliffs, New Jersey

woman's contemporary image

a personal and professional guide

Library of Congress Cataloging in Publication Data

Contemporary Programs, Inc.
  Woman's contemporary image.
    1. Beauty, Personal.   2. Etiquette for women.
I. Adams, Jean   II. Title.
RA778.C733 1975   646.7'02'4042   74-17367
ISBN   0-13-962274-8

WOMAN'S CONTEMPORARY IMAGE:
a personal and professional guide

Contemporary Programs, Inc.

© 1975 by Prentice-Hall, Inc., Englewood Cliffs, New Jersey

Printed in the United States of America

10   9   8   7   6   5   4   3   2   1

Illustrated by Ray Skibinski

Prentice-Hall International, Inc., London
Prentice-Hall of Australia, Pty. Ltd., Sydney
Prentice-Hall of Canada, Ltd., Toronto
Prentice-Hall of India Private Limited, New Delhi
Prentice-Hall of Japan, Inc., Tokyo

With gratitude and affection, we dedicate
WOMAN'S CONTEMPORARY IMAGE
to our families and business associates for their interest and help;
and to God who provided the inspiration
to complete our work.

contents

three
business image

preface

Today's contemporary scene reflects an era of rapid change, an age of shortcuts, and a time when leisurely living is almost nonexistant. Within this fast-paced social framework, the modern woman is expected to competently, efficiently, and with poise and self-confidence, progress toward her personal and professional goals. She must constantly accept new challenges that expand her mind and new modes and methods of dress and grooming that enhance her beauty. This new, vibrant, woman, whether her career is in the home or in the business world, wants to project an independent image that proves to the world that she can achieve a higher level of career professionalism, become more adept at good grooming, and enhance her ability to get along with other people.

Contemporary Programs, Inc. (CPI) has worked with banks, corporations, colleges, and women's groups to help today's woman discover the fun way to look and feel a part of what's happening *now*. Through prestige personal improvement courses at conventions, colleges, and businesses, CPI has helped many women create a new look of elegance. Not just appearance and grooming alone, however important they may be, but by successfully teaching the art of an attractive total image: appearance, voice, social intelligence, poise, and professional behavior.

National surveys and a series of personal interviews were conducted by CPI with business and professional men and women throughout the country. Executives at all levels of management answered detailed questionnaires, expressing their opinions on the characteristics and traits that they considered essential for a successful woman employee to have. Their answers are reflected in the complete professional and personal improvement course that is brought to you in this book.

For information regarding seminars write:
Contemporary Programs, Inc.
P.O. Box 25101
Houston, Texas 77005

one

individual
image

how to be a liberated woman and remain feminine*

It is not necessary to discard one of woman's strongest attributes—her femininity—as she emerges into the working world. The Emerging Woman's Guidelines that follow are a key to seeking one's independence and *remaining* feminine.

The Women's Liberation Movement (Women's Lib), with its large impact on contemporary lifestyles, has made both women and men aware of woman's struggle for independence. Now that the early struggle is past, thoughtful solutions that include both sexes are being sought. Men and women are struggling for purpose and independence and seeking lifestyle changes to permit this. Man will no longer be under intense pressure to perform as sole provider. Woman will not be destined or obligated to be a dependent domestic. Roles may be shared rather than preordained by virtue of sex, and more options will be opened for the individual. The young will grow up with more realistic insight into their parents because both parents will more equally participate in their upbringing.

The key to achievement in this new world centers around education, perseverance, setting goals, willingness to make personal sacrifices, desire to succeed, sensitivity to others' needs, and understanding of the mutual role of men and women.

Is it necessary for a woman to discard her femininity as she

---

*The development of ideas for this chapter began in the book by Martin and Jean Adams, *The Emerging Couple* (New York: Dell, 1973).

emerges? Of course not. Those who have done so have found the going rough, and their effectiveness as individuals has been diminished. Being feminine is not being a man's plaything. Being feminine is retaining those qualities that imbue confidence, grace, and poise in a world of men and women, enhancing our self-respect and our effectiveness as individuals. The Emerging Woman's Guidelines provide an outline for independence *and* femininity.

THE EMERGING WOMAN'S GUIDELINES

Education. Whether or not education is gained formally with certificates and degrees to back it up, being an informed individual is essential to growth. Unless one knows what options are available, how can a rational, informed choice be made? Ignorance is the antithesis of being informed, and decisions based upon ignorance are completely open to chance—things may turn out right, or they may not.

By obtaining and completing her formal education, the young woman keeps important options regarding her lifestyle open. Unfortunately, too many young women in the past failed to complete their educations formally for various reasons, the leading cause being that they were moonstruck and "in love." This decision often led immediately to marriage and a future destined to dependency, economic and otherwise. Ten years later, many of these women awake, endowed with families and working husbands, finding themselves unfulfilled and bound within roles they are expected to fulfill. They never knew other choices in life, and whatever latent capacities for enrichment they may have possessed previously have been dulled. Their options at this point of awakening are especially difficult, for lifestyles and living patterns have already been molded and are difficult to change.

Completing degree work is no absolute insurance that this hazard can be avoided. The choice really is up to the individual. However, by developing marketable skills and the self-confidence that comes from accomplishment, the young woman can make a *wiser* choice about how she wants to live and with whom, if anybody, she wants to live.

Independence is, in a very real way, intertwined with personal economics; that is, people have to be capable of buying or otherwise affording their own independence. This obviously requires that they have something of value to sell in the market place. Degree training is one of the most important pathways to attaining this objective. But it bears repeating that this is no guarantee. For one thing, obstacles to career growth still exist in many organizations that may employ one's skills. These will not disappear overnight; only unrealistic women believe they will.

A different and more intelligent way of looking at the question of education for women is to think in terms of careers instead of degrees. Recent surveys have shown, for example, that husbands look much more favorably on careers for their wives than nine-to-five jobs. The *career*, however, was perceived to be purposeful, useful, respectable, and, importantly, nonconflicting with husband's own ego needs. What are these careers that husbands and younger men find rewarding for their women? The list is long, and it includes medicine; psychiatry; accounting; law; business requiring decision-making such as fashion, sales, and advertising; research; and academic fields other

FIGURE 1.
The CPI owner-directors. Left to right, front row: Lou Davis; Maggie McDonald, executive vice president-secretary. Left to right, back row: Betti Saunders; Dorie Damuth, president; Eva Farley, treasurer; Maxine Breed, assistant secretary-treasurer; Jean Adams, chairman of the board; Sidney Faust.

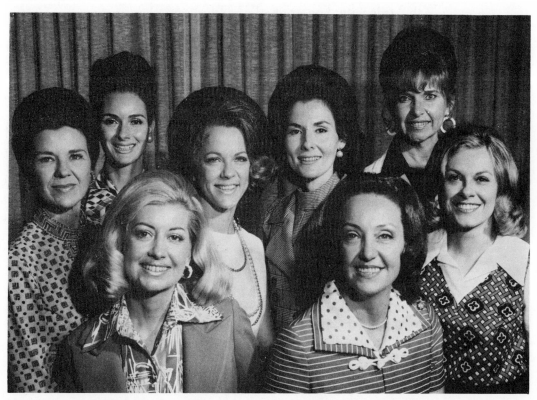

than the usual elementary school teaching. Men, in other words, voiced their approval of fields of endeavor for women *outside* those which were held by women in the past. The CPI stockholders, for example, combine the roles of housewife, mother, and career woman. (See Figure 1.)

If, then, people think in terms of careers for women instead of jobs, teacher certificates, and the like, then let them borrow another page from man's book and think in terms of entrepreneurial effort. How many women in America have been recognized "entrepreneurs?" Not many. When they did pursue activities outside the home, they were most often somebody else's "help-mate" and were employed by organizations that were originally conceived and created by men. They too can be entrepreneurs, creating profit-making organizations that fill a niche in business or society, and enjoy the same kind of economic and emotional rewards that men have enjoyed in the past. For example, they can and should develop their own profit-making entities as well as demanding that large corporations open career opportunities at the top for women. The needs are many, if women just look about them.

Perhaps female activists have been too busy complaining about the status quo and not really doing anything about it. For example, the franchise boom of the sixties saw the emergence of many so-called "fast food" service chains, selling everything from hamburgers to fried chicken. Many survived the economic shake-out of the late sixties and went on to become prosperous enterprises in the seventies. Although the kitchen has been considered woman's province for many years, hardly any female entrepreneurs are to be found among the ranks of the *nouveau riche* who made it big in the food business. This is preposterous, considering that women fried chicken over hot stoves and grilled hamburgers for their families long before anybody ever heard of the Kentucky Colonel. *Women must do less complaining and more doing if they are to make substantial contributions to themselves and to society in the future.*

One area that is ripe for female entrepreneurial activity is the entire gamut of child care. By working out the means of caring for the young, if it is possible to do so profitably without sacrificing quality and competence, emergence and independence will become a reality for many women who only dream of it now. If women fail to develop workable solutions in this important sphere, they can be assured that more ambitious males will develop them instead, and another opportunity under their noses will be lost.

This is but one opportunity for women to work, contribute, and utilize every ounce of their educations. There are many others for women who want to do things "the American way," which has always been the way of the entrepreneur. Large, successful, profit-making organizations didn't just happen—they were usually developed by a single individual (admittedly usually male) with an idea and persistence. Women, through application of their educations and experience, can and should accomplish the same, not envying those institutions that man built, but learning from them.

Why should woman's formal education cease when her first degree is attained? If she has truly digested the concept of "career thinking" instead of job preparation, there is no reason at all for her to stop. The first degree can open many doors to more specialized and advanced study. By the time her first degree has been completed, she will have a better idea about a career. Even some diagnostic aptitude testing at this point could be helpful in order to highlight her strongest skills and aptitudes, aligning these with various career fields. This can be enlightening, too, because she might discover that she now has aptitudes for fields of specialization she had never dreamed of.

Scholarships, part-time work, and summer jobs can all make further study possible. Unthinkable as it may first appear, loans on very satisfactory terms can be negotiated from banks and other sources for this purpose. There is nothing really new about these techniques for financing higher education—men have done it for years. They often complete their educations owing large sums of money to lenders and go on to repay these loans over a period of years so that the money can be re-lent to others in the same situation, and the cycle continues. At first, the lender may be skeptical about providing funds to a young woman because she is still *supposed* to be economically dependent on her husband. With success, however, this skepticism will die away, and the way will be paved for others.

It was mentioned earlier that a formal education leading to a degree is not the only education. Alternative to this, the woman who knows what she wants can take specialized course work in professional or technical fields and still achieve her ultimate independence. If, for example, she chooses computer programming, fashion design, interior decorating, real estate, insurance sales, or art (and the list of choices is multitudinous), real fulfillment can be found in developing skills in this way. A B.S. or B.A. degree is not the only pathway to fulfillment. Involvement, commitment, purpose, dedication, and contribution are the elements that can enrich a life and give it meaning and direction. The world's needs are growing increasingly larger with complexity and population; the result is that there is a need somewhere that each person can fill.

Perseverance. To persevere is literally to cut right through to the heart of the matter: This is what it takes to be a liberated woman, yet one who is feminine. Women live their lives not by being like every other person, but by maintaining and amplifying their uniqueness, by preserving their individuality, and above all by knowing who they are and where they are going. This might seem selfish. It is. But unless a woman considers herself first and does the most she can with the way she looks and acts, she may have little to offer others. If women are happy, dynamic, satisfied individuals, their radiance will spill over to others and will bring joy to their lives. Individuals can do this only by knowing what is going on inside themselves, observing situations, people, and opportunities around them, and by using their talents. This requires that they set goals in their lives, whatever those goals may be, and that they be not easily manipulated or dissuaded from their attainment. People are what they are—in their looks, dress, manner, and actions. They should not be apologetic or remorseful about their uniqueness. Persons are not to be hung up about these things. Indira Ghandi once said, "There are two kinds of people, those who do the work and those who take the credit. I would rather be in the first group because there is far less competition there."

This is perseverance: setting goals and following through.

Setting Goals. Goal setting is a technique that has been utilized successfully in man's world for years. Practically all modern businesses are geared around goal-setting. This concept has equal pertinence for women's personal lives. Important as it is, the goals that people set for themselves must be realistic. Nothing is more frustrating than to set unrealistic goals that cannot be attained no matter how hard one tries. In order to be realistic, facts are required, not daydreams. These facts include knowledge about one's self: capability, skills, personality, and capacities as well as personal likes and dislikes. In addition, people need to know the facts, as well as they can be presented, about the situation toward which they are planning.

The best goal-setting methods involve timetables. When does a person want to reach a certain point? What events must take place in order for her to reach that point? Is it reasonable to expect that she will, in terms of her time, talent, energy, and resources? Goal-setting usually begins with questions of this type. Some are difficult to answer because they assume that people know themselves and what they want to achieve. Such knowledge is especially elusive in young people. But goals should not, and must not, be inflexible. Situations change and people change, revising their goals many times throughout life. It will help you to begin with these questions:

1. What goal or goals do I ultimately want, as a person and as a woman?
2. What training, preparation, and experience do I need to reach these ultimate goals?
3. How can I acquire this training, preparation, and experience?
4. Am I willing to make the sacrifices that may be necessary?
5. Are my ultimate goals realistic in terms of my abilities, capacities, and limitations?

Having thought about these questions, it helps to list them and write out the answers on paper. You should write and rewrite them until you are satisfied that you are saying what you mean and being completely honest with yourself.

You may want to discuss your answers in a give-and-take discussion with someone in whom you have confidence. Diagnostic aptitude testing at this point, as previously mentioned, can help you to check further. Keep the option open to modify these preliminary goals if there is a need to. Then, begin to develop a timetable that ultimately leads to your goals, and set about meeting it. But a word of caution: One should not make goals so inflexible that they cannot be changed. Life is full of surprises, and some of these surprises may actually boost one toward reaching these goals.

Willingness To Make Personal Sacrifices. Almost any goal worth attaining requires sacrifice. Most of us don't really like the idea of sacrifice because it requires compromise in the sense of giving up, at least temporarily, indulgences or pleasures we may actually prefer. If it is more comforting to think in terms of compromise than sacrifice, fine. Still, there is no escaping the need to be willing and able to select between alternative courses of action in a balanced way. Some proponents of Women's Lib recommend abandoning their families in order to be completely free of any necessity to make compromise. In certain extreme cases this might be a recommended route, but for most people it is pure nonsense. Few people desire such complete freedom or are so selfish that they require such extreme courses of action. Most are sensible and patient enough to grow while maintaining the worthwhile things in life and working out compromises for the others.

Being liberated but feminine requires this sort of dedication to the principle of compromise. If women, in becoming liberated, lose their femininity, it soon becomes obvious from their appearance and manner that they want what they want *now*, with little regard for the feelings and sensitivities of others. It is axiomatic that women with families, seeking various degrees of liberation while retaining their femininity, *must* be willing to compromise. There is no other way. Even the ordinary demands of family living in conventional marriages, but especially liberated ones, require compromise.

Certainly at this point it is reasonable to ask, "Why compromise at all? Doesn't this slow one down in reaching those goals that were discussed earlier?" Really, the choice is whether or not a liberated woman wants to live in close proximity to other people. Give-and-take compromise is necessary even in living with or among other liberated women, but especially when living with men. Some people develop lifestyles that require few compromises. Usually these people require little close companionship with either sex. Some are perfectly content to live this way. Others require more companionship, even the companionship that marriage can provide. So the choice is individual, depending on needs, likes, and dislikes.

Many women find that it is impossible to be an effective wife-mother-career person, fashionplate, and entertainer, all at the same time. Most families still believe that while children are young, mother's place is in the home. This certainly is true *if* family members are unwilling to compromise by sharing larger responsibilities than they might otherwise. A dedication to the principle of compromise in many cases has made it possible for the wife-mother to continue her career uninterrupted, like her husband.

If one requires the companionship of others on a continuing basis, then the give and take of compromise can actually accelerate the attaining of certain goals and objectives. This occurs naturally, because others appreciate sensible compromise and become supportive. Contrast this with the uncompromising, never swerving personality who insists on having things only her way and in her own time; this person antagonizes and creates obstacles that can impede her progress.

So far, the only compromises discussed involve those with human situations. Compromises with things or events, sometimes beyond control, are just as important. For example, one might have the urge to drop everything for two or three weeks and take a pleasure trip, fully knowing that this could seriously jeopardize certain essential projects. What can be done? Maybe a compromise can be worked out that would involve only a three-day weekend trip for now, while planning something more extensive later on. This is an example of compromise. One is often tempted by side excursions that simply aren't realistic at the time. Compromising gives one *some* of what she wants at a particular time, holding out more for later.

People in pursuit of demanding goals, career or otherwise, often find little or no time for hobbies or other diversions. This, too, is an example of compromise, but it borders more on *sacrifice* than compromise. Sacrifice, the act of literally giving something up in the interest of attaining goals, should be avoided if certain things or activities are important in one's life. You may be too tired, for example, to attend church on Sunday morning, preferring to sleep instead. Yet, if church is important to you, it might be best to get a little more sleep on Saturday night. If church really isn't an important part of your life, then you might decide to skip it. Most choices about the importance of certain things and activities are personal anyway. Clearly, if *all* things and *all* activities are equally important, then it will be impossible to compromise and will only lead to frustration.

Compromise is being willing to give in—but not to give up!

Desire To Succeed. Desire is probably the most important guideline in this chapter. Desire, persistence, and perseverance all rolled into one can overcome many obstacles and can even compensate for otherwise serious shortcomings. For example, intense desire to earn a Ph.D. in literature and become a college professor can compensate for a lack of funds or even a physical handicap. With a great enough desire, one finds ways around these obstacles.

If one lacks the desire that is necessary to succeed in some endeavor, she discovers it soon enough and eventually *gives up*. The principle of compromise that has been discussed might seem to some that a temporary loss of desire is recommended. This is certainly not intended. Desire transcends compromise. One might have to make temporary adjustments or compromises, but the desire to reach the goal must continue.

A fifty-three-year-old woman was widowed after thirty-six years of marriage. Many years had passed since this woman had earned a teacher's certificate after two years of training at a small college in Louisiana. Determined to resume teaching activities, she returned to college and after two years of course work and dorm mother activities, she became an English literature teacher in a high school. She gave herself fully to this newfound career. Preparation for classwork was difficult at first, requiring several hours of work each night, often involving grading papers and essays between five and seven a.m. Yet she wanted to do the best job she could and to give her students the finest college preparation they could receive. This year, only two months before her retirement, she was awarded a "Lifetime for Youth" award at the Future Teachers Association state convention in Dallas. She had been designated an outstanding teacher by all who knew her, and students honored her because she gave them the only true gift: herself. This honor was especially meaningful as she was the choice of a statewide conference of student leaders. Fifteen years ago, this woman could not have envisioned such attainment. Desire made it possible.

Sensitivity To Others' Needs. Often, self must come first. But there are ways to put self first and still be considerate of the needs and feelings of others. Some of these methods were discussed in the section on compromise and sacrifice. A well-known writer had a friend who often came calling at four p.m. Frequently, this conflicted with the writer's thought processes and work schedule. But this was a good friend, otherwise thoughtful, considerate, and interesting to be with. The friend usually wanted to discuss something that, to her, was important. The writer realized this, and because she valued this friendship, listened. Sometimes she had been tempted to brush her friend aside. But this would have hurt both of them. Finally, because the writer was unselfish with her time, the friend settled the matter on her mind, and the afternoon visits soon disappeared. The situation worked itself out naturally, and neither person was hurt. Had the visits continued to interfere, the writer could have compromised by readjusting her schedule; she could have confronted the situation directly by telling this friend that she was interrupting important work; or she could have refused to see her friend entirely. In this case, being sensitive to the needs of a friend paid off. It usually does.

Should woman be expected to possess such empathetic qualities in greater abundance than man? No! Successful men know that sensitivity to others—warmth, sincerity, empathy—are presumed to be womanly traits. Nothing could be more farfetched. By having sensitivity to others' needs and conveying it, these same qualities return many times over.

The Mutual Role of Men and Women. In the past, men have felt threatened by the antics of liberated women (or those becoming liberated). Resentment grew in men because their dominance was challenged; women retaliated because they believed men were unreceptive. People have been confused by the polarity of the sexes and have decided that a more realistic appraisal of roles is in order.

If woman is to succeed in a world that has long been man's province, she must realize that he still expects most of the same prerogatives he has enjoyed in the past. This is not to suggest that these expectations should be tolerated without reason, or indefinitely. Just be mindful that they do exist and that they do, to a large extent, regulate the attitudes and behavior of most adult males. In this relationship with men, woman's biggest hurdle is to *win his respect*. To do this one must conduct herself responsibly, ably, competently, and sincerely. She must be as professional in her field as any man can be. She must react to adversity or frustration without bursting into tears or resorting to other mind-bending, emotional tactics simply because "women are supposed to behave that way." In brief, she must *surprise* man with her responsible behavior.

Women who elicit this kind of approval from men are *confident* in themselves and in their abilities. They expect to be treated as equals, and they are fully capable of backing it up. If, for whatever particular reason, it means letting the man wear the pants, these women can do so without feeling deprived or abused. There are times when a situation calls for woman to wear the pants. She does so without malice, without deflating male ego, without lording it over him.

Man learns to *trust* this woman. His experience shows that he can trust her to be more competent in some situations than he can be, still letting him retain his dignity. She does it by being feminine and human while she is also liberated.

ENRICHMENT ACTIVITIES

1. Choose one Women's Liberation leader who appears to be feminine and prepare a short report on what she does or does not do that makes her that way.

2. List the traits that you believe a liberated but feminine woman possesses and compare these traits with your own.

3. Conduct a poll among men to find out how they feel about the liberated woman; find out what they think a woman could do to remain feminine as she gains new freedom in this world. This poll can be turned into an exciting short report on the attitudes of today's men.

4. Observe and learn to classify types of male-female relationships. You can do this by observing the behavior of your friends or other couples. Is the male domineering and the female passive? Or, do they tend to share equally in a give-and-take behaviorial pattern? In what areas is one or the other more aggressive?

2

the sound
of you

"For it is by this one gift that we are most distinguished from brute animals, that we can converse together and can express our thoughts," Cicero wrote.

Speech is a gift that can be used fully and effectively, yet the majority of people never take advantage of all the inner equipment nature bestowed for the production of speech.

Women are perhaps the guiltiest of all creatures in this respect. A vast amount of time and money is spent polishing, painting, and garbing the visible you, but indifference settles like a cloud when it comes to the idea of improving one's speech or communication. You may shrug your shoulders and declare, "I've talked this way since I was born. I can't change!" One major fallacy behind this statement is that you were not born talking! You *were* born with the equipment for producing voice and speech. How you use it or abuse it is up to you. Caring about its use is the first step toward change.

Are you aware of how quickly you are judged by your voice and speech, at least on first contact? Think back to the times you have formed an opinion of someone by his or her voice, particularly over the telephone. Just as a dog responds to the qualities in a human's voice, so do people. Even in the theatre, certain voice characteristics are equated with personality types—the strident tones of the shrew, the boisterous sound of the bully, or the sultry note of the vamp. Disraeli said, "There is no index of character so sure as the voice." Your voice should stay in step with your personality and reflect the best of you. No one expects you to project the pear-shaped tones and pure diction of great actresses who have devoted their lives to such training. Yet you can strive to develop a voice that is pleasant, natural, relaxed, enthusiastic, void of ugly, discordant sounds, and one that radiates the best of your personality. If you consider that some of the greatest speakers in history, such as Demosthenes and Churchill, overcame speech handicaps, you, too, may try to improve toward more attractive communication.

Being aware of how you should sound to others is a major step in the right direction. It is important to first understand the mechanical working of speech, and then it's up to you to oil the machinery.

An important step is to listen *objectively* to your own voice. When a person hears herself for the first time on a tape recorder, she usually suffers mixed emotions. She may be both fascinated and appalled. The tape recorder is a revealing vocal mirror, and all the blemishes show. Because of its honesty, it is by far the best way to develop a pleasant speaking voice. If you don't own a tape recorder, then try cupping your hands over your ears and speak a few sentences. Being aware and caring how you sound to others is the first rung on the ladder to successful communication.

THE PRODUCTION OF SPEECH

Next, learn how voice and speech are produced. When the breath is exhaled, it passes over the vocal cords or folds, causing them to vibrate. (See Figure 2.) The sound is transformed into speech by the *articulators*—the lips, teeth, tongue, and hard and soft palates. The *resonators*—the sinuses, nose, mouth, chest, head, and throat—act as amplifiers, giving the sound *resonance*.

The richness, depth, and projection of the voice is dependent on correct breathing. Most women are shallow breathers. Your shoulders should not rise up and down when you talk. Place your hand on your chest, say a few phrases, and see if your hand moves.

To breathe properly, concentrate on the lower part of your body, the abdomen or diaphragm. The *diaphragm*, a muscle located between your chest and the abdomen, is the main muscle used in breathing, as illustrated in Figure 3. It gives the necessary support to your breath, which in turn supports your voice. Activate the

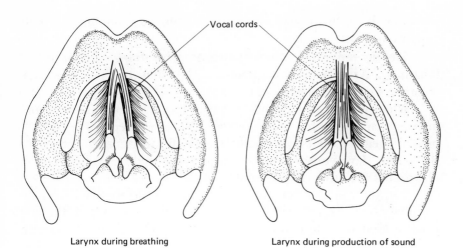

Larynx during breathing   Larynx during production of sound

FIGURE 2.
When the breath is exhaled, it passes over the vocal cords, causing them to vibrate.

diaphragm by placing your hand on your diaphragm, and pant like a dog. Holding your shoulders down, open your mouth and breathe in and out, concentrating on the center of your body. Try taking a deep breath, holding it, and slowly exhaling, controlling the output. Pretend you are a flat tire, s-l-o-w-l-y going flat. The object of these

1. Sinus
2. Nasal cavity
3. Hard palate
4. Soft palate
5. Lips
6. Teeth
7. Uvula
8. Tongue
9. Pharnyx
10. Epiglottis
11. Vocal cords
12. Windpipe
13. Lungs
14. Diaphragm in repose
15. Diaphragm in inhalation

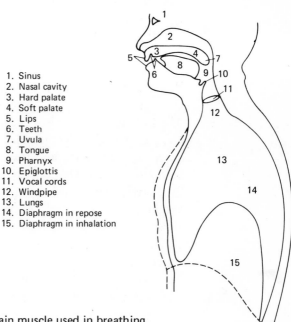

FIGURE 3.
The diaphragm is the main muscle used in breathing.

exercises is to help you locate the diaphragm and put it to its supportive use.

The desired goal is not so much deep breathing, but *controlled* breathing. After you have practiced the "flat tire" exercise, try counting on the exhaled breath.

When you heard yourself over the tape recorder, did you sound higher than you felt you talked? Most women do speak in high-pitched voices; unfortunately, the greater the tension, the higher the pitch. Have you noticed that when you become excited, angry, or irritated the pitch rises upward?

Tension can also cause unpleasant vocal qualities such as a raspy or nasal voice. To relieve tension, try yawning or slowly rolling the head around from left to right with the eyes closed and the mouth open.

For pitch, count up and down the scale just as you would vocalize. Find a comfortable pitch that is right for you; however, do concentrate on the lower range, particularly when you are working with your recorder. Learn to control your pitch with the emotional climate at hand.

The major vocal faults lie in four categories: the nasal voice, the harsh voice, the breathy voice, and the baby or immature voice. All result from using the equipment of speech incorrectly.

If you detect nasality in your voice, it may result from lazy lips and tongue. Sound cannot come forth if you barely open your mouth. Look at yourself in the mirror and see how you talk. Tight lips and jaws will produce a nasal sound.

A harsh voice can come from weak support and a forced voice. Practice the exercises for support and tension.

Breathy voices occur when the outgoing air is not controlled; The flat tire exercise is recommended for this problem.

A "baby" voice, which many girls think is cute, does not impart sense or confidence and loses its charm with each year. Direct your attention to vocal support to overcome this habit.

Articulation is the production of sound into recognizable symbols. Each sound is produced in a different way. You can sharpen your articulation by working with tongue twisters or by placing a toothpick or a kitchen match between your teeth for exercise.

To achieve good diction, you must beware of the pitfalls of faulty grammar, slang, carelessness, or colloquialisms.

1. Give words their full value. Don't leave off the endings of words such as "goin," "thinkin," "gol" (gold).
2. Don't run words and phrases together such as "cancha," "wudja," "couldja."
3. Don't add sounds to words. For example, "warsh," "Warshington," "umberella," "mischeevious."
4. Don't overwork certain words or phrases such as "you know," "and everything."
5. Do take the time to pick up a book on speech and learn more about this subject.

Your gift of communication is a precious thing and should be tuned constantly as you would a fine musical instrument.

TELEPHONE TALK

The telephone is a great timesaving device. Our social and business life is so geared that everyone has a tendency to take the telephone for granted. Therefore, it is valuable to occasionally reexamine our attitudes and use of this instrument.

Whether for social or business reasons, you project your image over the phone sight unseen. The listener can only interpret your meaning by your voice and speech. He cannot see how attractive you look, nor can he see the smile on your face.

When you use the phone in daily conversation, you should keep these points in mind.

1. The way you answer the phone, your "hello," can tell the caller many things about your mood—whether you are up or down, busy or bored, glad or sad. Answer the phone with a warm "hello," the same way you'd greet someone in person.
2. Don't go into a vocal slump over the telephone. Speak clearly, with warmth and vitality.
3. Be considerate when you call someone at home. Don't go into lengthy chatter without asking, "Are you busy?" or, "Am I interrupting?" Remember that when you initiate the call, social convention places the responsibility on you to conclude it.

Although your friends will forgive your telephone inadequacies, this is not true in business, where your job and your company's image depend on your telephone tactics. How you answer the phone and handle various situations is of the utmost importance. You become a symbol—a salesman, a representative, an ambassador—for your company or boss. Many people judge a firm by the way calls are received. It takes all the tact, patience, and courtesy one can muster to cope daily with the phone. Still, it is your job and you must strive to do it well.

Here are some "do's" and "don'ts" for building public relations via the wires:

1. When you answer the phone, identify your company, your department, or give your name. Never answer with an indifferent "hello."

2. Answer the phone with confidence. Convey a message of goodwill and a sincere desire to help. Try to use a low-pitched voice. It seems to help create a mental picture of authority and business. Never assume an artificial, affected manner.

3. Speak clearly into the mouthpiece. Don't chew gum, smoke, or gnaw a pencil.

4. Don't pick up the receiver while engaged in conversation with someone in the office. Finish one conversation before starting another.

5. Keep a pad and pencil by the telephone ready for you to jot down messages.

6. Learn to identify names. This will build your company's image. To go even further, you may become friendly with some clients or customers. People enjoy being recognized. Calls with these people must be governed, however, so that they do not become lengthy conversations.

7. Listen attentively to the caller's request. If you must transfer his call, be sure you understand his business, ask his permission, and then try to connect him with the *right* department. There is nothing more frustrating than being sent from one department to another.

8. If you must put someone on "hold," check back frequently. Never keep them in suspense, wondering if they have been forgotten or are holding a dead line.

9. When you are a secretary for a busy executive, you should receive calls in the manner *he* prefers. If he is busy and asks not to be interrupted, never ask the caller's name and *then* announce that he is busy. Also, there's something chilling about an abrupt, "Who's calling?" A little padding, such as "*May* I ask who is calling, *please*?" is much less offensive.

10. When you are responsible for placing calls, prepare yourself beforehand with all the necessary information. Take the time for a little mental rehearsal so that you make your request in an intelligent, efficient manner.

11. Keep all files, information, and business data at your fingertips.

12. When conversations are concluded, leave a good impression lingering behind you. A pleasant "Good-bye," "Please call again," "We are happy to help you," will work for you and your company.

THE ART OF CONVERSATION

It is often said that conversation is a lost art; the culprit that usually shoulders the blame is television. Yet it hardly seems fair to fault a media of communication that brings timely news, entertainment, and education right into the living room. Perhaps the blame rests more on people who do not examine their attitudes toward this "art." Some rules of conversation remain as solid today as they have for decades, while other areas have changed, just as basic rules of etiquette have altered. The art of conversation is based on the quality of courtesy and consideration for others as well as one's own self-confidence.

First, consider how courtesy and consideration for others play important roles in making a good conversationalist. Books on conversation emphasize *being a good listener* and *taking an interest in others.* Think about the following:

1. Do you really take an interest in other people's thoughts, experiences, and opinions? When you feel at a loss for something to say, do you try to find an area of interest to encourage the other person to talk? Do you ask them questions that will encourage and stimulate *their* thinking?

2. Do you really listen? Or, do you let your mind stray, planning what you're going to talk about next (hoping they'll finish quickly so you can dive in!)? Do you let your *eyes* wander around the room? Do you assume a glazed, vacant stare (an obvious giveaway to your disinterest)?

As for conversational courtesies, regard these thoughts:

1. Do you monopolize conversation, never giving others a chance to talk? Do you suffer from "I-trouble," letting *I* dominate your sentences? What about the other pronouns, *we* and *you*?

2. Do you keep people hanging while you snap your fingers trying to recall a name or date? Move on if it isn't relevant to your story. Don't bore your listeners with too many minute details.

3. Do you interrupt someone's conversation with a pointless remark or question, or, worse, to argue a point? This is a sure way to kill their enthusiasm. Above all, don't steal someone else's story, even if you think you can relate it better.

4. Instead of being concerned with your own shyness, look around for the person who is even less confident and try to draw him out, particularly at a social gathering.

5. Don't ask questions that invade one's privacy. Learn to be sensitive to other people's feelings, and avoid areas that are *none of your business*.

6. Benjamin Franklin said, "I speak ill of no man and all the good of everybody." It's a good quote to remember when talk turns to gossip. "People talk" is a normal conversational gambit, but when it is malicious, harmful, and destructive, it should be eliminated. It may work against you, making others distrustful of *you* as a friend.

Having "talkable" topics for conversation is a necessity. They can only come from your interest in the world around you. Certain topics were at one time labeled taboo—sex, religion, and politics. As times have changed, attitudes have become more tolerant, and there is no reason to shun such thought-provoking topics. Retain your "sensitivity antennae" so that you neither embarrass nor hurt someone with your opinions. Try to discuss topics objectively without the heat of anger or personal prejudice.

Read newspapers, books, and magazines to stay abreast of the world happenings in entertainment, education, world problems, sports, politics, personalities, and so on. Don't let television limit your conversation, but, rather, let it enhance it. Let your vocabulary grow, not stagnate. New words will not enrich your vocabulary if you merely look up their definitions in the dictionary. You must understand them, learn their usage, and *use* them.

Participate in life. Not only should you read and listen, but *do*. Your own experiences will work for you by making you a more interesting person.

You can also make a lasting impression with the way you *look* and *sound* when you talk. Be careful about nervous mannerisms such as twisting your hair or playing with objects on the table. Hands should be used gracefully to make points and as a means of description. It isn't necessary for them to lie lifelessly in your lap. On the other hand, they should not flail the air constantly, upsetting the nearest glass or bric-a-brac.

Look directly at people when you are talking to them. If you are in a group, include everyone in your conversation. Speak with warmth and enthusiasm, just as a salesman would to sell a product he believes in. After all, in conversation you are selling yourself, whether through your kindness, your courtesy, your stimulating ideas, or your pleasing personality. Sell the very best You!

PLATFORM POISE

It is rare that a person can move through life without being confronted by some public speaking experience—in clubs, church, school, or business. It is amazing how many individuals, even hardened businessmen, quake at the thought of standing before an audience.

Stage fright can be so overwhelming that most people will dodge any situation that puts them in the predicament of delivering a speech. Actually, stage fright can be useful. It can stimulate you and make you more alert. It should not conquer you. The majority of speech students in class suffer varying degrees of stage fright. Through practice and experience, they learn to *control* their fears. There may always be the anticipation and the nervousness at the beginning of a speech, but it should not be totally devastating. Eleanor Roosevelt said, "I believe that anyone can conquer fear by doing the things he fears to do, provided he keeps doing them until he gets a record of successful experiences behind him." With confidence gained through practice, each moment becomes easier. This is why everyone, if possible, should take a speech course. Not everyone has the opportunity to study public speaking; the following rules are listed to help any novice.

1. Always evaluate your audience, their age, number, occupational and educational backgrounds, and interests.

2. Prepare your speech. Preparation is the key to self-assurance.

3. Practice! Get the feel of your voice and your material. It may be helpful to practice before a mirror or to tape your speech.

4. Develop a natural conversational style. Do not read to your audience unless you want to read them to sleep. Nor should you memorize your talk. Speeches that are either read or memorized have a mechanical ring. Many speakers use notes or outlines. If you feel too insecure to use this method, then practice your manuscript until you know the text well enough to need only an occasional glance.

5. Approach the platform, stage, or podium confidently. Act confident even if you don't feel it inside! Don't rush your introduction, but take your time to arrange your notes, adjust the microphone, and do whatever is necessary to feel organized.

6. Don't begin with an apology, telling your audience, "I'm not a speaker."

7. Try to use eye contact. It comes with experience and is a must for reaching your audience. The goal is to make each person feel that you are speaking to him.

8. Take a deep breath, look your audience over, and *smile*.

> ## ENRICHMENT ACTIVITIES

1. Practice using a tape recorder to read passages that contain power and special meaning. Here are some examples:

   a. "God grant that not only the love of liberty but a thorough knowledge of the rights of man may pervade all the nations of the earth, so that a philosopher may set his feet anywhere on its surface and say 'This is my country.' "
   — Benjamin Franklin

   b. "We seek an open world—open to ideas, open to the exchange of goods and people, a world in which no people, great or small, will live in angry isolation. We cannot expect to make everyone our friend, but we can try to make no one our enemy."
   — Richard Nixon

   c. "Let our object be our country, our whole country, and nothing but our country. And by the blessing of God, may that country itself become a vast and splendid monument, not of oppression and terror, but of wisdom, peace, and liberty, upon which the world may gaze with admiration forever."
   — Daniel Webster

   d. "I have nothing to offer but blood, toil, tears, and sweat—You ask, what is our policy? I will say, it is to wage war, by sea, land, and air with all our might and with all the strength that God can give us; to wage war against a monstrous tyranny, never surpassed in the dark, lamentable catalogue of human crime. That is our policy. You ask, what is our aim? I can answer in one word; it is victory, victory at all costs, victory in spite of terror, victory however long and hard the road may be; for without victory there is no survival."
   — Winston Churchill

2. Make a list of frequently mispronounced words. Consult a speech textbook for a guide.

3. After taping your voice write an analysis of your voice based on the following:

   a. vocal appeal   pleasant

                                     annoying

b. quality	breathy	
	nasal	
	hoarse	
	resonant	
c. pitch	high	
	medium	
	low	
d. articulation	clear	
	not clear	
e. vocal effectiveness	monotonous	
	flexible	

4. Decide, as a result of your vocal analysis, what exercises would benefit you.

5. Interview business people about their opinions regarding telephone usage, complaints, and preferences.

6. Work with a partner, improvising various telephone situations.

7. Act out examples of both good and bad social conversations.

8. Research famous personalities and their experiences with stage fright.

9. Deliver a short talk about your stage fright and the experiences you have had facing an audience.

10. Demonstrate walking to the front of the room and assuming a correct speaker's stance.

    a. Walk slowly to the podium.

    b. Pause and look your audience over.

    c. Make a brief opening statement.

    d. Return to your chair.

11. Introduce a classmate. Include in your talk:

    a. His name

    b. His background information

    c. His interests (hobbies, travels, pet peeves, and future plans)

    d. A closing statement

12. Deliver a short sales talk and demonstrate a product to your audience. Use one of the following products:

    a. Household cleaners

    b. Electrical appliances

    c. Gadgets

     d. Make-up

     e. Sporting equipment

13. Prepare a short talk and deliver it to the class. Suggested topics:

     You Can't Buy Peace

     A Rebel at Heart

     Those Were the Good Old Days

     An Unforgettable Pet

     My Most Frightening Moment

     My Most Embarrassing Moment

     A Funny Thing Happened

     The Meaning of Friendship

     It Was a First

     A Strange Moment

14. Select a well-known quotation or proverb. Prepare a short speech, applying it to a modern theme.

3

social intelligence

One must not only know the rules of behavior but also practice those rules so naturally that those about her are continually asking, "What is her secret?" Such a person has an excellent inner image and has learned the social graces that make people relax and enjoy her on all occasions, ranging from a rap session at the office to a formal dinner.

Your inner image is conveyed in countless ways to those about you. Even in life's complex whirl, people are still aware of others; and they judge a person's image by her actions: by the way she walks, holds her head, speaks, or by the way she meets and entertains people. A perceptive person may readily learn another person's self-concept by observation. Recognizing that outer behavior reflects the inner image, one should exercise prudence in the way she does everything. For these reasons, social intelligence is a prerequisite to becoming a total person.

As more couples adapt to relaxed and informal living patterns, not all the traditional rules governing the social graces may apply. These rules may need to be altered in order to remain pertinent. Even so, it is important to be reminded of some of the rules so that they can be interpreted for today.

The woman with social intelligence recognizes that there are some social conventions that one should still respect even though the old rules have been modified. Furthermore, she provides herself with a book on etiquette, such as those by Emily Post[1] and Amy Vanderbilt.[2] She learns and practices the correct way. She must be knowledgeable if she is to be prepared for the demands of encountering people and if she is to maintain that charisma that sets her apart. How can you develop this social intelligence?

HOSPITALITY

First and foremost, you must be hospitable and practice charity and liberality. A warm, benevolent hostess can welcome her guests with an enthusiasm and interest that makes every person feel he is a VIP. The magnetism of the hostess motivates the guest, and his enthusiastic reaction continues to stimulate the hostess. Such interaction results in a hospitable hostess and a popular guest. Hospitality embodies more than friendliness and cheerfulness; a good hostess respects the eccentricities of those she entertains, whether they are peers or crackpots. If you do not know your guests well, direct conversation into channels that may reveal likes and dislikes of the one or group you are entertaining. To be hospitable, one must, indeed, be gracious. To attain the ultimate in grace and charm a woman must arm herself with intelligence, sagacity, and wisdom. A good hostess must know the rules before she can change them to meet her needs.

In addition to the normal rules that apply to social behavior, a few common sense suggestions are in order for the thoughtful guest. They are:

1. *Respond* to invitations. Let the host/hostess know whether or not you can accept their invitation. As a matter of common courtesy, always try to be positive in responding to an invitation. Nothing frustrates the hostess more than the "wishy-washy" person who is indefinite about plans to attend.

2. If it is your first visit, it is thoughtful (though not necessary) to bring a small gift such as candy, flowers, or a special beverage. A thoughtful gesture at any time is to

[1] Emily Post (Revised by Elizabeth L. Post), *Etiquette*, 12th edition (New York: Funk and Wagnalls, 1969).

[2] Amy Vanderbilt, *Etiquette* (Garden City: Doubleday, 1972).

bring a small remembrance for the children of the host/hostess.

3. Be considerate of other guests.

4. If alcoholic beverages are served, do not overindulge.

5. A good rule is to leave the party while things are on a high plane. Late stayers, seemingly insensitive to the lateness of the hour, often place the otherwise gracious hostess in the position of having to yawn, glance at the clock, or signal some other way to suggest that the party is over.

If you are the hostess instead of the guest, remember that a warm welcome and warm good-bye are special touches that make a

FIGURE 4.
The contemporary dinner party is often a relaxed affair with an atmosphere that can be attained on a limited budget.

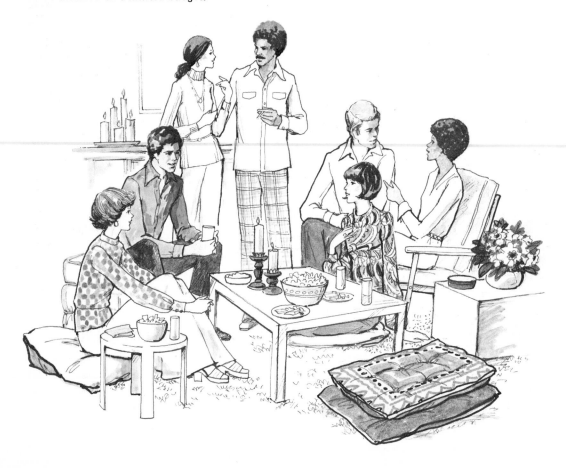

guest happy. An especially nice gesture by the hostess is to say, "Thank you for coming," as the guest departs.

Regardless of all the rules pertaining to social intelligence, the ultimate objective of every hostess is to ensure that guests enjoy the event. The most beautifully and properly executed occasion can be spoiled by stiffness, ritual, or boring conversation. How can you determine the social success of a party or special occasion? One effective way is by the comments you hear from guests. But a more reliable sign is that the hostess enjoys herself so much she practically forgets it is her party! (See Figure 4.)

At a New Year's Eve party recently the hostess greeted all her guests warmly as they arrived. She or her husband-host, whoever was available, arranged proper introductions among guests as they arrived. It was a large party, and some guests had known one another before. Actually, this was helpful because guests saw to it, as they mingled, that strangers were properly introduced if the host or hostess was not nearby. Beverages were served by a waiter, and later a buffet-style dinner was provided. As the evening passed, guests became caught up in their own momentum. They had beverages when they wished, and if the waiter was not nearby, they simply served themselves. The buffet-style dinner also made it possible for guests to serve themselves easily. Thus, there were few administrative demands made on the host and hostess after they had done their part to get the evening started. The guests did the rest! After the first hour, both host and hostess were so involved in interesting conversation with guests that they virtually forgot themselves. They enjoyed the New Year's Eve party at least as much as their guests—maybe even more!

You do not have to have a large party with waiters to create a relaxed environment for guests—it can be done for two to ten people if you do your homework before the guests arrive and relax in the casual environment you have created once they are there.

TABLE MANNERS

Because Americans eat on almost all occasions, one should know the rules for both informal and formal meals.

It has been said that the fellowships when eating surpass those enjoyed at any other time. Consequently, a hostess should be thoroughly relaxed and know that she has learned the rules.

For example, if you are having a formal dinner, you should not be disturbed that you have not seated the guests properly. By consulting the proper source, a correct hostess has learned the following seating arrangement for an informal dinner: The guest of honor, if a man, is seated at the right of the hostess (if a woman, at the right of the host); all others are seated according to rank, in descending order. If one does not have an official rank, his business position or financial status may be the determining factor. Assuming the guests are about the same age and of equal rank, *Vogue's Book of Etiquette*[3] gives the following order: a guest invited to a meal for the first time, a stranger, a holder of important position in the past, a guest who has been present before, guests who are frequent visitors, house guests, relatives, and children of the household. The host, seated at the head of the table, is usually near the entrance of the room, and the hostess at the opposite side (end) is near the entrance of the area from which the food is served.

Excellent seating charts for official and unofficial dinners are found in Emily Post's *Etiquette.* Knowing the rules of seating people, today's host or hostess is free to make the changes necessary for a delightful meal for her guests. One must often make changes in table precedence to have a congenial, happy group. Today, much important business is transacted at the most informal dinners, where hostesses vary the rules to meet their needs. (More and more businessmen prefer informal entertaining to the more formal atmosphere of "cold chicken banquets.") These same hostesses would, no doubt, consult an authority for a very formal dinner. Such a minor thing as the seating of guests need not disturb a hostess if she has access to all the necessary information.

Another facet of dining that disturbs people is the use of silver. The order has been the same for many years: the silver that is used last is nearest the plate. If the salad course is first, the salad fork is placed before the dinner fork. The steak knife is used in place of a dinner knife if steak is served. Teaspoons are not put on the table unless they are to be used for bouillon or cream soup. The iced tea spoon is to the right of the knife. (Naturally, the menu determines the silver to be used.)

[3] Millicent Fenwick, *Vogue's Book of Etiquette* (New York: Simon and Schuster), pp. 325-26.

Modern hosts and hostesses vary these rules; but if you are having a formal dinner, you can quickly learn by consulting etiquette books with excellent illustrations and rules governing table settings. Whether she is right or wrong in her placing of the goblet at the end of the knife should not concern a hostess; she should know the correct way. If she wants to do it differently, she should do what pleases her. The point is that a good hostess is comfortable and relaxed at all times. If you choose to place the napkin at the left of the silver or in a new fold on the plate, feel confident about the way you have done it, and forget it.

Difficult foods may be a problem for a hostess who wants to spend her time with her guests. Casseroles and meat dishes that may be prepared before dinner relieve the hostess of last-minute tasks that might be frustrating as she tries to welcome her guests. If the hostess has no help, she should by all means plan a menu that permits her to relax and enjoy the dinner. Women who enjoy serving food should continually add to their recipe files foods that can be quickly or easily prepared and foods that can be prepared before guests arrive. Today's markets offer a great variety of food that help the busy woman.

Dining in the home may be as elaborate or as simple as the home can afford and the hostess wishes. More and more, the informal meal at home is the choice of a good hostess. There are many reasons for choosing a dinner at home. First, a guest may feel the hostess is most appreciative of him if he is invited into the privacy of the home. Also, if the hostess wants to use a unique mode of service, she has the freedom of her home. By far, the most important advantage of a meal at home is the intimacy it affords family and friends. The genuine fellowship in a home cannot be equaled. The memory of a beautiful meal shared in the home lingers with both hostess and guest long after they part.

Dining at home is not always possible or reasonable. Often, people must take their guests to dinner at public places. Here again, some simple rules should govern the choice of the restaurant or eating place. If you know your guest well and know what food he enjoys, you may find it easy to decide where to eat. Surely a considerate hostess would never take a guest who dislikes cafeterias to a cafeteria. Again, if children are a part of the group, a good hostess is mindful of them and their needs, choosing a place where children are comfortable.

Another matter of social intelligence that concerns the hostess is the proper way to make introductions. Emily Post's *Etiquette* (pp. 1-14) gives the rules of introduction as follows:

1. A younger person is presented to an older person. "Mrs. Jones, may I introduce you to Miss Smith."
2. A gentleman is always presented to a lady even though she is no older than eighteen.
3. No woman is ever presented to a man unless he is the President, recognized head of another country, member of royal family, or a cardinal or church dignitary.

Other rules of introduction, using Emily Post's *Etiquette* as a guide, are as follows:

1. The simplest form is the mere pronouncing of both names: "Mrs. Keats, Mrs. Johns"; or if a man and woman are being introduced, "Mrs. Grant, Mr. Judd."
2. "Mrs. Brown, my stepfather Mr. Jones." is a rule that many want to know. Remember that the preposition *to* makes a difference in introductions. A woman's name must be said before a man's unless *to* is used, for example, "Mr. Jones, may I introduce you to my daughter Susie?" If Susie is married, add her last name. In addition to these, an introduction of wife or husband is very important; and it can be very warm. The inflection of the voice says as much as the words. Friends are close, and John may say to them, "I want you to meet my wife." (He never says "the wife," "the boss," or "the madam.") He then may add his wife's name.

Teenagers and young adults are less formal, and the casual "Hello" is acceptable. People can be less formal, as in asking "John, do you know Alice?" or adding a favorable comment about the one they are introducing.

If the hostess remains in the presence of the newly introduced parties, participating in their conversation for awhile, there are some points for her to bear in mind that are perhaps more important than the rules of introduction. She should politely steer the conversation away from matters pertaining to the usual: "Well, what business are you in?" "Where did you grow up?" "Did you attend high school in Wichita?" "How many children do you have?" Certainly if the guests are interesting human beings, there can be more to discuss than these trite queries.

At a dinner party attended by fourteen guests who were not previously acquainted, the hostess introduced two of the men to each other, in the proper manner. She knew that each was an interesting person in his own right. Feeling comfortable with the introductions, she left them alone and went to check on how things were progressing in the kitchen. One of the two, unfortunately, began the usual rhetoric—"who, what, when, where"—obviously seeking identity and trying to determine just how he might categorize his newly made acquaintance.

After a few of these questions, the second man suddenly responded, "Look, let me tell you about myself so you won't have to ask. I'm a gigolo and my wife is a multimillionairess. She supports me, so you might say I'm a kept man. I've been married six times before and I have twelve children. I was born in this town and attended high school and college here. I have a notorious reputation. Now if you'll excuse me." And he promptly left the first man standing, wondering what had hit him. Although the second man was not behaving as a thoughtful guest should, he is an excellent example of one who is fed up with trite conversationalists and expects more from a social gathering. Obviously this situation is more extreme than most. However, it is an example of the kind of unpleasantness that can happen.

Men often become aggravated when women can discuss nothing but their children, garden club, bridge club, or church group. Women—and men, too—become annoyed at the man whose entire world consists of his business career and can discuss nothing else. In conversation, people often tend to place far too much emphasis on a man's business affiliations so that they can sketch a mental picture of his "type"—rich, famous, powerful, artistic, creative, generous, technical, and so forth. By doing this, people are subconsciously reassuring themselves by concluding, "Oh, yes, he's just like these other people I know."

Another dinner party was attended by a group of famous and near-famous people. The party was hosted by a man and his wife who functioned as agents for several of the guests. It was a small, informal affair with an attendance of eighteen. Although none of the guests had met before, one could spot a few familiar faces, perhaps because of television appearances or magazine pictures. After introductions were made, the guests enjoyed a truly delightful evening because topics of conversation never retreated into the usual, trite line of typecasting questions. Conversations dealt, instead, with such matters as politics, religion, art, gourmet foods, current books—almost any subject of broad interest.

Even if guests have never met one another before, they can spend an entire evening together in interesting conversation that never resorts to "who, what, when, where." It is a temptation to begin an acquaintance by trying to categorize each other this way. Perhaps this is human nature. Or, more likely people simply feel more comfortable once they believe themselves to be familiar with a new person or a new situation.

For a truly refreshing experience when you are introduced to someone new at a social event, let the conversation deal with topics about which you have ideas and would enjoy sharing with another person. If all goes well, you may discover that you can fruitfully spend the entire evening without playing "who, what, when, where." Then, if you are curious about the occupation, fame, or fortunes of the other person, ask someone later on—or do a little research yourself! Often one can learn a lot about another person as fascinating topics are discussed.

Social intelligence—why is it important? If you are to be "in the know" in this space age filled with excitement and adventure, there is no time for doubt and error. When you know the rules and choose to break them, you are then in control of the situation. It was Ogden Nash who broke the rules in writing poetry, and he said that he could break them because he knew them. Every hostess should know what she is doing, and her ingenuity should allow her to make changes that make her more charming.

TIPPING

Tipping has become a "must" in the American way of life if one is to have the best service. Fifteen percent of a bill is considered a correct tip for service at the table or in the hotel room. Unless the gratuity is added to the bill for the food, the tip is expected. Often, room service has an additional charge and the tip is still necessary. Tipping is not in order for hotel managers, but thoughtful permanent guests or guests of long periods remember desk clerks with gifts. To know the exact rules of tipping in hotels, on ship board, in airplane travel, in beauty parlors, for cabs, and various other services, read rules for tipping found in authoritative etiquette books.

SMOKING

Smoking is another item of concern in social intelligence. Few people consider the proper time to smoke. Of course a lady does not walk down the street with a cigarette in her mouth; never is she that indiscreet. If she ignores the reports of the possible injury of smoking, she should know some rules concerning smokers. Always she adheres to the "No Smoking" sign on buses, streetcars, and trains unless she is in the area where smoking is permitted. A considerate person never smokes in a nursery or sickroom unless those who are there are smoking and a cigarette or cigar is offered. Many businesses have rules that govern smoking; one should know these rules and the rules that govern public places, such as museums, theaters, and courtrooms.

Furthermore, if you smoke, you should know how to handle your cigarette. A lady is never conspicuous in the way she holds her cigarette or exhales the smoke. She is very careful to leave the butt in the ash tray; and if she chooses to put it into a garbage can, she makes certain there is no fire by holding the cigarette under water and wrapping it in paper before dropping it into the container. If you choose to smoke a cigar, these rules still hold, and you should remember not to talk while the cigar is in your mouth. You should watch the ashes to be sure they do not fall on furniture or rugs. Never light or let another light a cigarette unless it is supported by two fingers—never should it be lit while hanging from the mouth. In our contemporary society of liberated women, a woman should carry her own matches and feel comfortable lighting her own cigarette if necessary. Again, common sense and discretion dictate that a person be considerate of others. A smoker should not bring discomfort to those about her.

Most of the so-called rules prescribed for proper social behavior were originally based on the notion of masculine dominance and feminine passivity. As new, more liberated lifestyles continue to develop, these rules will naturally evolve to fit the circumstances. More than half of all women in America over sixteen years of age have jobs and careers, and the percentage is increasing. Rules that were originally intended to protect man's place may become less important in the future. The real measure of the quality of a person is the person herself.

ENRICHMENT ACTIVITIES

1. Plan a critique dinner party: Invite several close friends, preferably couples, over for dinner and do everything perfectly that night—have food, table service, and other matters all in order according to proper etiquette rules. At the end of the evening, ask guests to criticize the evening, giving their comments, both pro and con. The guests should be informed of what has been done. This exercise is most effective done with close friends who will be honest.

2. Discuss social graces through a question-and-answer game. Divide into two groups and keep score on etiquette IQ as the game progresses. Use a complete etiquette guide, such as *Vogue's Book of Etiquette*, to gather extra question information and as source material for correct answers. For example, one question might be: Where does a female guest sit at dinner when she and her husband are the only guests of another couple? Or, is it always correct to present a man to a woman when introducing them? One member of the class might be assigned the duty of looking up questions to be used and serving as scorekeeper. Perhaps the teacher would like to do this. In any event, this type of exercise is best performed with other classmates; friends might not be so cognizant of social graces.

3. Take a poll of people under twenty-five to find out what they feel proper etiquette in modern society should be. Most young people do not practice extremely proper etiquette today, and it might be interesting to discover what they think social graces should be. These questions can be derived from the same book used in the preceding exercise. Women's Liberation

should become apparent in this poll if questions like the following are asked:

a. Should a man walk on the outside?

b. Should a woman wait for a man to light her cigarette?

c. Should a man wait for a woman to get off an elevator before leaving, himself?

d. At a large table, do you feel everyone should wait to begin eating until all have been served their plates and been seated?

If enough people are interviewed, the poll will include sufficient statistics to write an interesting short report, giving both the facts and a few comments from the interviewees.

two

visible
image

haircare and spare hair

YOUR HAIR AND ITS CARE

Healthy hair is beautiful, lustrous hair. Make a habit of the four basic elements of hair care: cleanliness, stimulation, restoration, and protection, recommended by doctors, dermatologists, and cosmetologists.

Hair does not have bounce and shine unless it is clean. Stimulating the scalp by brushing and massaging helps to keep hair and scalp in top condition. If there is a scalp problem or excessive loss of hair, it is advisable to see a dermatologist. Don't abuse your hair; protect it from harsh environmental elements, excessive bleaching, too many permanents, and everyday abuse.

According to national surveys conducted by CPI, eighty-six percent of the businessmen and women and college students listed hair as the first physical feature of women noticed by them. According to personnel and training directors, there are three major hair problems among women employees that confront all companies. *The major complaint is unclean and unkempt hair.* The other two grievances are elaborate "after-five" hair styles worn to work and long hair hanging down over the face. Company executives want their women employees to have clean, shiny, healthy hair in a natural, becoming hairstyle.

MAKE IT SHINE AND TINGLE

Brushing. With a brush of good natural bristle, get into the habit of giving your hair a thorough daily brushing. A good brushing

43

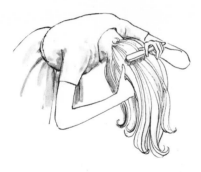

FIGURE 5.
A daily brushing routine helps keep the hair and scalp in top condition.

routine, as illustrated in Figure 5, cleanses, airs and stimulates. It also distributes beneficial oils, removes dead skin cells and loose hair, and gives life to curls.

Invest in a good boar bristle brush—soft bristles for baby fine and tinted hair, stiff bristles for wiry and thick hair. The bristle tufts should have a slight, loose separation so they will penetrate the hair strands.

Don't count. Just brush until the scalp tingles. Brush in sections. Start at the bottom and work up until the hair is free of tangles. Then, slightly touching the scalp, use long, firm strokes out to the very tip. Be careful not to twist or snap the brush at the ends as this will cause the ends to split and break. Bending at the waist, lean forward and brush the back hair forward over the head. Then in an upward position, brush hair from front to back. To really get into the swing, alternate two brushes, one in each hand.

To avoid transferring dirt and oil from one section to the next, stop at intervals and wipe the bristles with a clean cloth. If you have oily hair, wrap the brush in cheesecloth or pack wads of cotton between the bristles to absorb oil and grime. To help eliminate electricity, wrap the brush in a nylon stocking. (The bristles will penetrate the nylon.)

If the hair is weak or damaged, excessive brushing is not recommended. Gently brush hair to remove tangles, and spend more time on scalp massage to improve and increase circulation.

Always keep your brushes and combs clean.

Combing. Tortoise-shell combs are best for everyday grooming. A comb with a combination of fine and coarse teeth is for average texture hair. For thin and fine hair, choose a fine-tooth comb; coarse teeth will help to tame thick or wiry tresses. Rattail combs can be used to give a lift to a hairstyle, and a teasing comb of staggered rows of long and short teeth helps to abolish extra hair breakage.

Massaging. Many women ask, "Why a scalp massage?" It increases the circulation of the blood that carries vital nutrients to feed the scalp and helps to relieve nervous tension. A nervous disorder can result in dry, lifeless hair as well as loss of hair.

Women also ask, "How often should you massage?" At least three times a week for ten minutes, but preferably three to five minutes each day. How can you massage? Using both hands, slide all ten fingers under your hair, then with the pads (not your nails) of your fingers slowly rotate the scalp in small, circular motions. Begin at the nape of the neck, work your way up the back of your head, over the top to your temple. Then starting behind your ears, work along the sides of your head. Massage until every inch of your scalp tingles.

KEEP IT CLEAN

Shampooing. One of the most important things women, or men, can do for their hair is to keep it clean. The most-asked question about clean hair is, "How often do I shampoo?" As often as needed, once or twice a week or even every day, but always frequently enough to keep the scalp free of scale and oil. (See Figure 6.)

Many believe that washing the hair too often causes the scalp and hair to develop a dry, dull condition. According to dermatologists, shampooing not only relieves dry dandruff but makes the scalp oilier rather than drier. Dullness is caused by accumulated dirt and oil.

Before shampooing, brush your hair to eliminate surface dirt, tangles, and hairspray. When you shampoo, wash your hair twice: the

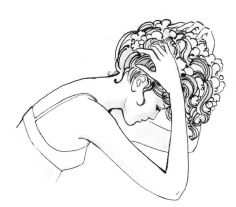

FIGURE 6.
Shampoo as often as necessary to keep the scalp free of scales and oil.

first sudsing to eliminate dirt and excess oil, the second sudsing to really get it clean. Always shampoo and rinse with warm or tepid (never hot) water.

Another question often asked is, "How do I shampoo my hair correctly?" The most important thing to remember is that wet hair loses natural strength and breaks easily, so give it tender, loving care. Begin your shampoo by wetting your hair thoroughly with lukewarm water. Pour a shampoo product labeled for your type of hair into the palm of your hand and work it into a lather. Then give your scalp a massage treatment with the pads of your fingers. Do not pull or twist the hair strands as this causes tangles and breakage. Rinse thoroughly. Rinse until it's squeaky clean. Then rinse with cool water to close the pores of the hair cuticles. Gently squeeze and blot out excess water with a towel; then comb or brush. Do not forget to shampoo your combs, brushes, curlers, clippies, and so on. They should be as clean as your freshly shampooed hair.

There are many types of rinses to give your hair additional body, manageability and sheen, and to dissolve soap curds from the hair after shampooing. If frequent shampooing is necessary because of an oily or scaly scalp, be careful that the rinse you use does not leave a film of waxy fat, necessitating additional shampooing.

Conditioners. There are conditioning treatments designed to add body to thin limp hair; help make coarse hair more manageable; add sheen to dull, lifeless hair; prevent snarling; and reduce electricity.

Dry, brittle, and abused tresses need the benefits of such conditioning treatments as the hot oil treatment. Thoroughly apply warm olive oil, castor oil, or a vegetable oil to the scalp. Follow with a heat cap or a succession of towels wrung out in hot water. If possible, let hair soak in the oil overnight.

KEEP IT HEALTHY

The ideal head of hair has an abundance of life, luster, and shimmery elasticity with enough body for easy management. The condition and type of hair you have are governed by many things: heredity, glandular and hormone changes, environment, nervous tension, menstruation, pregnancy, illness, medication, external treatment, improper diet, lack of sleep, overexposure to sun and wind, and other abuses.

If you have ideal hair, or if that is your goal, remember the four basic elements of hair care: cleanliness, stimulation, restoration, and protection. Because your hair is a barometer of your health, you need to maintain a well-balanced diet, a calm disposition, and a good health routine.

Start by analyzing your hair. What is its present condition? Is it dry, normal, oily? Is it fine, wiry, coarse, or curly, and is it tinted, flaked, or abused? Are the ends split and broken and the texture like straw?

If you are suffering from an excessive loss of hair, flaking, or badly damaged hair, *never* self-treat or ignore it. These disorders need the prompt attention of your doctor or dermatologist. Without prompt, proper treatment, these can lead to more serious complications, including baldness. And who wants to be a baldheaded lady?

Coarse or fine and curly or straight hair is an hereditary gift. Take advantage of these in your hairstyle.

Coarse Hair. Coarse and wiry hair is usually dry and needs lots of brushing and massaging to stimulate and distribute natural oils. Luxuriate in hot oil treatments and crème conditioners to insure against brittleness.

Expert shaping is the key to success. Use a heavy setting lotion and gently stretch the hair over extra large rollers. After the comb-out, spray with extra-hold hairspray.

Fine Hair. Fine hair is usually on the fragile, thin side. It either hangs limp from humidity and summer heat or flies away with static electricity in the winter. You need a soft, loose permanent for body; frequent shampooing and setting with super-hold waving lotion, gel, or stale (undiluted) beer for more bulk; frequent hot oil treatments for vitality; extra-hold hairspray for control; brushing and scalp massage for stimulation; and a protein or crème rinse for manageability.

Because long hair pulls out waves and is hard to control, keep your hairstyle short, perhaps layered, so that it will not weigh itself down. Use either medium or small rollers, and brush your fresh setting carefully.

Curly Hair. Curly hair is a blessing and a curse. It is great not having to spend time, money, and effort for hair curl, but curly hair limits hairstyles, tangles easily, and develops "humidity kinks." The easiest answer is to stop fighting the inevitable and have the hair shaped in a style that takes advantage of the curl; a professional cut with the curl in a short, soft style gives a lovely appearance that needs a minimum of care.

To reduce curl, use a heavy waving lotion or gel; as you set the hair with large rollers, gently stretch the hair. Brush out carefully so as not to undo the set, and spray with extra-hold hairspray.

A good electric comb or brush that blows warm air as it combs can help to keep the hair straight. Remember that electric combs and brushes are drying, so condition your hair to counteract the dryness and try not to use the electric comb or brush daily.

Fashionable blacks find freedom in braiding (cornrowing) and in the "natural" or "Afro" style. The "Afro" is very attractive for many women but needs careful proportioning to body frame and facial features.

For those who want to try straight hair, there is the straightening permanent.

Oily Hair. Oily hair can be caused by dandruff, by a diet that is too rich in fats and oils, by infrequent stimulation, and by improper shampooing.

Wash the hair frequently, and this may mean daily. Be sure all shampoo is removed by using a rinse such as lemon or vinegar. For emergencies, you may use a spray or powder-type shampoo, baby powder, or cornmeal to remove excess oil and grime. Extra stimulation by brushing and scalp manipulation will help to regulate oil glands.

Because of frequent shampooing, a short, simple hairstyle will be the easiest to manage. Use large rollers rather than small ones as oily hair has a tendency to separate.

Dry Hair. Dry hair may be the result of a poor diet, mental or physical strain, or lack of needed treatment. Good nutrition, high in natural fats and protein, and lots of care will help to restore healthy, shiny hair. Stimulate blood circulation and oil glands with scalp massage and brushing. Brush and comb gently, as dry hair strands break easily. Avoid teasing, hot hairdryers, and excessive exposure to sun and wind. Condition with postshampoo crème rinses, protein conditioners, and preshampoo hot oil treatments. A hairstyle that needs little or no setting is preferable because dry hair is easily damaged by rollers and clippies.

Gray Hair. Because gray hair is usually wiry and dry, daily massage and brushing are extremely important; you need to increase the stimulation of oil glands and blood circulation. Use rich shampoos, rinses, and conditioners, and do not forget to treat yourself to hot oil treatments.

As you mature, you need to camouflage the facial muscles that begin to "sag." Do this with short, fluffy hairstyles or the hair softly lifted away from the face. As you are undergoing chemistry changes within your body, you will need to get the advice of your hairdresser about rinses; and if you want to color your gray, have it done by a professional.

Dandruff.   The shedding or flaking of scalp skin can be associated with either a dry or an oily scalp. Dry scalp conditions can be improved with daily brushing and massaging, correct diet, and frequent shampooing with an antidandruff shampoo, followed by a thorough rinsing. In this way, a healthy scalp can be encouraged and flakiness eliminated. An inexpensive recipe for removing dandruff and cleaning and stimulating the scalp is to apply equal parts of white vinegar and water to the scalp with cotton balls.

Excessive flaking of an oily nature accompanied by itching and red scalp patches can be harboring harmful bacteria that can spread to the eyebrows and face. Medical treatment is advisable because this type of dandruff can lead to loss of hair and skin complications.

Baldness. Baldness, ranging from total loss of hair to partial thinning, may be caused by heredity, aging, illness, nervous disorder, medication, scalp disease, or abuse. If you are experiencing a minimal loss of hair following surgery or illness, dermatologists suggest that you shampoo your hair frequently, massage your scalp daily, and maintain a well-balanced diet and health routine. During this period, you should have a hairstyle that does not need to be set, and you should avoid permanents and coloring.

COLOR YOURSELF NATURALLY

Modern haircoloring gives every woman an opportunity to be more attractive, to look younger, to enhance and maintain her natural beauty.

The two most-asked questions about haircoloring are, "How do I keep from damaging my hair?" and "How do I determine which color is right for me?"

Complexion, age, and personality must be taken into consideration for haircoloring. You should choose a color that is complimentary to your complexion tones; even with a slight change in color, it will be necessary to make changes in your makeup. As you mature, beware of fiery reds that give you an appearance of fading or black-browns and jet-blacks that harden a face. If you do not want the gray or salt-and-pepper look and want to go back to your original color, go two or three shades lighter for a more flattering and youthful look.

Before using any kind of haircolor, it is a must that your scalp and hair be in good condition. If you have had a permanent or your hair straightened, wait at least two weeks before any attempt at using a haircolor. And *never* color your eyelashes or eyebrows with either a temporary or permanent hair rinse or tint.

The three types of hair coloring are:

1. Temporary rinse or color—washes away with the next shampoo. It does not bring about major color changes but simply highlights your own color and shade.
2. Semipermanent color—emphasizes highlights in your color and shade. It gradually washes out, and a repeated application is needed in four to six weeks. You can go a shade darker or lighter than your original shade.
3. Permanent tints or dyes—liquid color agents that penetrate the hair shaft and change the pigment.
    a. In the one-step process, a developer or bleaching agent, which removes some of the natural color, is mixed with a tint, which immediately replaces the new color.
    b. In the two-step process, a lightener or bleach is applied, which penetrates the hair shaft and removes the pigmentation. Then a tint or toner is applied.

It is recommended that permanent hair tints be done by a professional. Cosmetologists know when to stop the bleaching process, how to apply tints or tones, the timing involved, and how to use two or more related colors to obtain the effect of a single color.

Frosting (hair strands lightened over various parts of the head), streaking (a lightened strand, usually at the front hairline), and tipping (wisps of hair lightened in various areas) do not have to be repeated as frequently as total hair bleaching and do not reach the scalp. Even though these processes are not as risky, it is advisable to have them done professionally.

ADD A WAVE OR SUBTRACT A CURL

A permanent wave, which lasts from four to six months, adds body to the hair and helps it to hold a set. Your choice of a permanent, either the salon or the home kit, should be determined by your hair type and texture. Invest in a professional permanent from a reputable salon if you have dry, brittle, gray, or tinted hair, or if you are uncertain about the outcome of your efforts.

If you have the ability and time for a home permanent, be sure to select the right hair fomula—regular for medium amount of curl, super for hard-to-wave, gentle for body, and specialized waves for gray and tinted tresses. Your hair must be in prime condition before you attempt a wave and, as you know, the manufacturer's instructions should be followed carefully.

Wiry and unruly curls can be tamed with a reverse permanent that will straighten the curl for approximately three months. The chemicals in a straightening permanent are the strongest and most damaging, and only hair in the best of health should undergo this process. After the waving lotion is applied, the hair is stretched and pulled with a comb. Too much combing can cause breakage, even partial baldness. As this is a risky process, it may be to your advantage to have your hair straightened by a professional.

SHAPING UP

Correct hair shaping is the foundation for well-designed hairstyles. The most skillful setting will not hide a bad cut. With a good hair shaping, the hair will retain a set longer, and as the set falls, the hair will still have a good design. The added bonus is a good cut that grows out gracefully.

You cannot do a good styling cut yourself. It must be done by a professional who can make your texture and type of hair look its best.

The Looks To Look For. There are several factors to be considered when deciding on a hairstyle: the shape of your face, the type and texture of your hair, your personality, size, and lifestyle.

For day wear, you need an easy to manage, neat, attractive style. The businesswoman's rule of thumb is that her hair hang no longer than shoulder length. To achieve the professional look for long hair, swirl it into a neat chignon or twist. If you are maturing, do not forget to "fight that sag" with a short fluffy hairstyle or a softly lifted twist or bun for long hair.

Before determining and deciding on your hairstyle, always remember that you are an individual—there is no one on earth exactly like you. Do not put yourself into a mold with your hairstyle. All shape faces can be beautiful. You do not want to be a "carbon copy;" you want to be an "original." Hairstyle camouflage is necessary only if you have an objectionable facial feature. Naturally, you want a style that minimizes your negative features and compliments your good features. Here are some suggestions that have worked well for women in CPI programs.

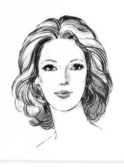
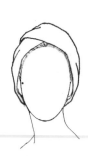

OVAL

The oval face, which is approximately one and a half times longer than the brow width with the forehead a little wider than the chin, is considered the most versatile shape—any coiffure may be chosen.

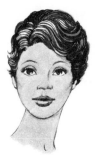
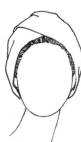

ROUND

Do: Keep hair fairly smooth and close at the sides. Try loose fluffiness, soft curls, or high waves at the crown.
Experiment with a slanted part.

Don't: Wear straight, low bangs.
Part your hair in the center.
Use round curls.

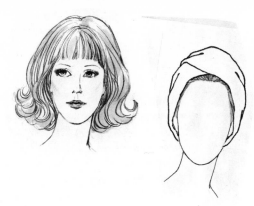

OBLONG

Do: Add fullness at the sides.
Shorten a high brow with fluffy bangs.
Try a side part.

Don't: Add additional height.
Wear straight, dangling hair.
Use a center part.

SQUARE

Do: Wear hair shorter or longer than jawline.
Add soft waves or curls at cheekbone.
Try a side part and soft, side bangs.

Don't: Pull your hair back at forehead.
Attempt straight-across bangs and straight line cut.
End your hairline at cheekbone.

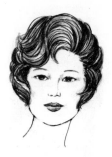
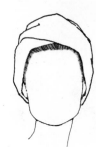

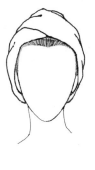
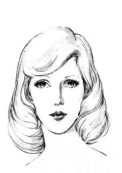

HEARTSHAPE

Do: Choose a soft, rounded coiffure that adds
fullness at the lower part of the face.
Extend the style into a pageboy or loose curls
below the ears.
Cover the forehead with soft bangs.

Don't: Wear styles that are swept back and high at
the crown.
Part your hair in the center.
End your hairline or hairstyles at ear level.

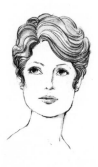
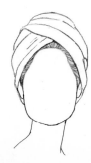

PEARSHAPE

Do: Add fullness across the top of your head.
Keep the hair smooth, pulled back, or short
around the sides.
Try a short hairdo that flows up in a cluster of
curls in the back.

Don't: Wear a style that has fullness at the jawline.
Part your hair in the center.
Subtract width at the temples with a hairstyle that
is smooth and flat.

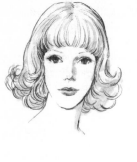
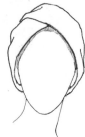

DIAMONDSHAPE

Do: Style your hair to add width at the temples.
Try soft, fluffy bangs.
Add width below the cheekbone with soft curls
or a pageboy.

Don't: Wear a center part.
Add width through the cheekbone.
Completely expose your forehead.

EYEGLASSES

Do: Try a rounded style that lifts away from the face.
Keep the sides simple.
Flip up ends slightly below the ears.

Don't: Add another facial feature with crowded bangs
and forward curls.

Camouflage Tricks. Here are some easy camouflage tricks with hair to help you improve your appearance.

Large Nose:	Keep front of hair soft and high. Avoid center parts.
Small Nose:	Use forward curls.
High Forehead:	Hide behind bangs.
Low Forehead:	Fluff hair away from face.
Receding Chin:	Lift hair to fluffy bangs and fluffy back curls.
Jutting Chin:	Add height at top and fullness at sides.
Double Chin:	Keep both your head and hair high, curls going upward.
Short Neck:	Hair short with upward sweep.
Long Neck:	Hair long enough to cover the neck.

The Basic Cut. The woman who likes to add variety to her life gets a good basic cut and set so that she can change her hairstyle with her moods. A basic shoulder length cut can be worked into a flip, soft waves, or a pageboy. It can be swirled into curls, a twist, or a chignon. The informal look can be the ponytail, the "Martha Washington," or the stringy "Gibson Girl."

Setting Techniques. With a good styling cut, you should be able to do the rest. Styles are created with rollers, pincurls, and a combination of the two. For a longer lasting set, wet your hair and apply either a setting lotion, gel, or stale, undiluted beer.

Rollers. If your preferred hairstyle needs height, use rollers. (See Figure 15.) Select the size rollers for the curl you desire—the larger the roller, the looser the curl.

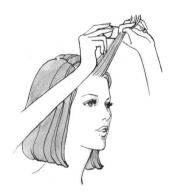
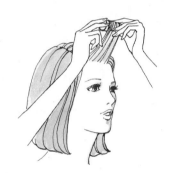

FIGURE 15.
Using rollers for height and lift.

Section off a strand of hair slightly narrower than the roller and approximately a quarter inch thick. After combing the hair section straight, gently stretch the hair up, wrap the ends neatly around the roller, and roll evenly to rest in the center of each section. The hair should be rolled in the direction you want the hairstyle brushed and combed. The rollers should be as close as possible so that there will be no separation in the finished coiffure. Secure with clippies. Note of caution: Never wind the rollers too tightly; remove them as soon as the hair is dry. Prolonged tension can cause hair damage and breakage. Never sleep in rollers; as you toss and turn during the night, you are pushing and pulling on your hair. This weakens, damages, and breaks the hair strands.

Pincurls. For bouncier, curlier curls, use pincurls. Section off a small block of hair about one inch square (larger for looser curls, smaller for tighter ones), and comb the hair section straight. Starting

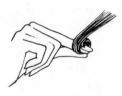

FIGURE 16.
The pincurl.

at the end of the strand, roll toward your face if it is to be a forward curl, away from your face if it is to be a backward curl. (See Figure 16.) The pincurl should be smooth, flat, and hollow at the center. Secure with a clippie. Producing good pincurls takes practice—and probably a little more practice—but the end result is worth the effort. As an aid, you can unravel a soft rope from knitting wool and roll it along with the hair.

Two or more rows of pincurls form a softer, fluffier effect. To produce a wave, alternate the direction in which each row is wound. For a pageboy, all pincurls should be rolled forward and under, changing the direction of pincurl slightly to one side of the back center of your head.

Hairdresser Tape. For hair worn short and straight in the back, a strip of tape placed across the ends will give a smoother, finished effect. Cheek curls and bangs can be secured with tape. For a direction to your bangs, comb to one side and secure. For bang height, after bangs have been combed in the desired direction, apply tape to ends and move upward to create a curve before attaching tape to the skin.

Electric Curlers. The mist type of electric curler is great for reviving wilted hairdos. Electric curlers may be drying and damaging to the hair, and it is recommended that they not be used excessively.

Blow Dryer. When blowing your freshly shampooed hair completely dry with a blow dryer, use a rubber-pronged or wire wig brush to style your hair. Brush and shape from a part in the crown, following the directions of the natural growth of the hair. Use warm air; hot air can dry and damage vulnerable ends and can actually scorch hair. Always brush and dry in long, even strokes from the scalp to the ends, remembering that wet hair has no elasticity and is easily broken. With a good cut, this blow dry and brush procedure should give you a soft, natural hairstyle.

Electric Curling Iron. The curling iron works best and is less damaging to dry hair. Never use the curling iron on sprayed hair: it will stick and may break the hair. The curling-iron hairstyle is meant to be loose and carefree.

Section the hair and insert the curling iron through a strand of hair approximately one-half to one inch from the scalp. Wrap the hair around the iron as you slowly and gently pull the iron out of the curl. If you start the curl from the end of the strand going toward the scalp, the curl will fall flat because the heat is at the end of the curling iron. The less hair that is caught in each strand, the easier it is to control and the tighter the curl will be. Always roll in the direction of the desired hairstyle. *Never* rest the curling iron on the scalp or keep the hair strand on the iron for a prolonged period. Let the curls cool before brushing or combing your hair.

The Comb-out. The comb-out is just as important to a hairstyle as the setting is. When the hair is thoroughly dry:

1. Gently remove rollers and clippies.
2. After a vigorous brushing, brush the hair in the direction you want the style to go.
3. If you need back-combing for body and line, begin teasing about an inch from the scalp.
4. To achieve a smooth finish, gently and lightly brush over the teasing.
5. With a styling lift, round out the hairstyle.
6. Brush and shape bangs, a curl, or wisps of hair to flatter the eyes and cheeks.
7. Mist the style with a water-soluble hairspray.

YOUR "SPARE" HAIR

Today's active and fashion-conscious women have discovered the versatility, convenience, practicality, and fun of wigs and hairpieces. For the career woman, they are proving indispensable, and many a businessman has found his second youth through a hairpiece. (Young men conceal their longer hair under wigs that give a more businesslike appearance.)

Company executives have no objections to employees wearing "extra hair" as long as they maintain a business image. The vice president of a national controls company said, "I like our women to be a blonde today, a redhead tomorrow. It adds spice to the old company."

A wig can conceal a multitude of sins. If a woman's hair needs washing and setting, she can slip into a freshly set hairdo. Deficient and damaged tresses can be hidden under the latest coiffure. Hairpieces can give short hair the illusion of length, add body to fine, limp, or thinning hair, and camouflage damaged or bedraggled hair. A woman can discover whether biondes, brunettes, brownettes, or redheads have more fun by a mere change of headdress.

THE POTPOURRI OF WIGS AND HAIRPIECES

Wigs offer a variety of colors, shades, styles, lengths, and proportions, as illustrated in Figure 17. The *full wig* may cover the hair completely or be worn with some of your hair combed into it. The *demi-wig* can completely cover the head or may be styled in a casual hairdo that covers a portion of the hair.

Hairpieces include wiglets, cascades, falls, switches, braids, curls, ponytails, and even pin-on bangs.

The *wiglet*, a flat-based hairpiece with fairly short hair, can be worked into the hair to give it height or body. It can be styled into curls or a chignon and attached at the crown or the nape of the neck.

The *cascade* has an oblong base that can be worn vertically with a style that goes from the crown to the nape of the neck or turned sideways to give width across the head.

The *long fall* (twenty to twenty-six inches long), the *wig fall* (sixteen to eighteen inches long), and the *mini-fall* (ten to sixteen inches long), can be worn either near or three to four inches from the

FIGURE 17.
Wigs and hairpieces, which can give you a new look and color change, are an essential part of today's fashion.

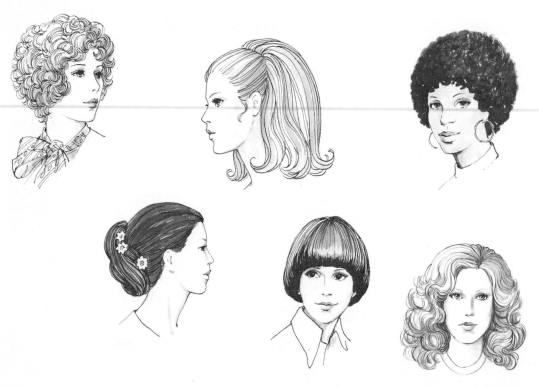

hairline. It can flow freely, be pulled back into a ponytail or chignon, or be styled in elaborate coiffures.

Switches, which vary in length, can be made into a chignon, braid, ponytail, french twist, or be coiled. The switch is as variable as your imagination.

Wigs and pieces can be made from human hair, animal hair, synthetic or man-made materials, or a blend.

The methods employed in attaching hair to a base or cap are hand-tying, wefting (machine sewing), or a combination of the two. The hand-tied wigs, usually a better fit and more natural looking, are lighter in weight; but because they are more delicate, they require more care. Custom-made wigs, which are the most expensive, are usually hand-tied. The wefted wig is less expensive, sturdier, and holds its shape better because the hair is sewn into the cap in circular rows. Hand-tied edges on a machine-made wig give overall durability of wefting and a more natural looking hairline.

BUYERS BEWARE

"What features should I consider when purchasing a wig or hairpiece?" is a question voiced at every CPI seminar. Many women feel that they have not received a quality wig or hairpiece for the amount of money they invested. As one woman summed it up, "I feel like I was 'took'!"

To protect the public from the effects of false labeling, advertising, and "swindlers," state and federal laws are becoming more rigid in the sale of "spare-time" hair. (By the early seventies, twenty-seven states required the licensing of people involved in the sale and handling of wigs and hairpieces.)

The quality of wigs and pieces is determined by the construction and the material used. The most important step is to buy from knowledgeable and reputable professionals who assure their services and guarantee their merchandise. They are specialists in their trade and know precisely what to look for in purchasing wigs and pieces. They are trained and have the experience to help you choose the most complimentary colors and styles. Why not take advantage of their know-how? As a double check, look for the following features:

1. The cap on a wig should fit close at the ears and nape of the neck, free of gathers. It should have a natural-looking

  hairline and be properly ventilated, durable, and comfortable.

2. The hair or fiber should be soft, lustrous, and natural looking; it will not have a nylon, coarse, frizzy, or brittle feel. Inferior hair and fibers have either a dull look or a glossy shine and pick up unnatural highlights.

3. Brush to determine if the hair and fibers are properly distributed and move easily in all directions. If the brush has an excessive amount of broken hair strands, look for another wig or hairpiece.

4. Check the top of the cap or base to make sure there are no bald spots, short protruding hairs, or swirls.

5. Machine stitching should be uniform with no loose threads.

6. A hairpiece should blend with your hair in color and texture. Otherwise, it will look false.

7. Be careful that a label reading one-hundred percent hair does not mean one-hundred percent animal hair.

WHAT WILL IT BE— HUMAN HAIR OR SYNTHETIC?

When synthetics were first introduced, they had an obviously "fake" look. Today it is sometimes impossible for experts to determine real from synthetic hair.

  The human hair can be mixed and matched to the exact blend of your own hair—or colored, tipped, streaked, or frosted. A temporary rinse can be applied to some synthetics to tone or highlight, but because the synthetic fibers are not porous, it is harder for the rinse to take.

  Human hair can be set and combed into different styles. The man-made fibers have their style baked in permanently; however, there are synthetics and blends that can be combed into different coiffures.

  European, Oriental, and a blend of the two are the three types of hair used in constructing human hair wigs and hairpieces. European hair is usually soft and fine while Oriental hair is of good body and texture, but usually coarse and straight. Some people prefer a blend of the two. Experts suggest that you purchase a wig or hairpiece with hair that has the texture and feel suitable for you and your needs.

Modacrylic fibers are considered to be one of the best synthetics. They are lightweight, have a natural luster, and good curl retention. They look and feel like human hair and in most instances do not change color when exposed to the sunlight.

Human hair must be reconditioned and will oxidize and fade when exposed to an excessive amount of sun. Rain and humid days may cause human hair to droop but has no effect on the artificial fibers. Human hair should never be permanent waved and should be cleaned in a wig-cleaning fluid. The man-made fibers are *wash and wear.*

Synthetics should not be exposed to a hot dryer, hot water, curling irons, or electric curlers. A blast of hot air from an oven can turn a soft curl into the "frizzies." Human hair can be damaged by a hot dryer, and because there are no natural oils and nutrients for protection, the hair strands can break from the heat of hot curling irons and electric curlers.

Synthetics and human hair can take gentle back-combing and teasing. An occasional light spray of a hairdressing helps eliminate dryness and a dull look. For hold power, use a water-soluble—never a lacquer—hairspray.

Many women ask CPI speakers their preference and recommendation as to human hair versus synthetic. The answer: The type that will be most beneficial to each individual according to her pocketbook, lifestyle, and capabilities in the grooming of "spare-time" hair.

WHAT ABOUT STYLING?

The two pet grievances expressed by businessmen and women about "part-time" hair are that it looks artificial on some women and that the women do not keep it neat.

Wigs and hairpieces create a frame for your face. Follow the same guide in their styling as you would for your natural hair. It is important that they be kept clean, neat, and freshly coiffured.

Synthetic and human hair wigs *must* be shaped and styled for you as an individual. To achieve the proportion for your facial structure and body frame, it may be necessary to thin and cut a substantial amount of hair from your wig. In other instances, it may require that a small amount be trimmed along the hairline. Do not be surprised if you have to make several trips to a wig stylist before you acquire the shape and style that is right for you. To enjoy the versatility of a human hair wig, it should not be cut to one style. You should be able to get at least three or four different coiffures so that you will not tire of the same look.

It is a requisite that your wig fit properly if it is to be comfortable and look its best on you. If the cap has shrunk through washing or if it has stretched through use, be sure to seek the help of a wigologist to solve the problem. A cap can be made smaller with a few darts or tucks, and most elasticized materials can be stretched.

The two areas that can be "tattlers," telling everyone that you are wearing a wig, are the *forehead hairline* and *around the ears.* Most wigs are styled with a bang of some type to conceal the unnatural look of the hairline. Fortunately, the majority of women can wear some version of a bang. If you prefer a sleek hairline, blend your own hair into the front of the wig. The area around the ears should be in a style flattering to your facial structure but should camouflage the earline.

With time, the baked-in styling of a synthetic will fall. Or, perhaps you have made the mistake of brushing or combing the curl out when your synthetic was wet. Do not throw the wig away; a wig stylist can give it a new look with a new style.

THE "HOW-TO" OF HANDLING WIGS AND HAIRPIECES

To go to a stylist for assistance each time you want to wear a wig or hairpiece can be expensive in both time and money. With a little practice—and lots of patience—you can don and doff your spare hair in minutes without disturbing the style.

If your wigs and hairpieces do not have small combs sewn to the front of the foundations, you need to purchase some griptooth combs and sew them in with a heavy thread, using a buttonhole stitch. Before donning your wig or hairpiece, make a large pincurl out of a section of your hair where the "extra hair" is to be attached. Fasten the curl with two or more bobby pins that cross each other. This will make an anchor into which you can slipe the comb of your wig or hairpiece. After the "extra hair" has been positioned, insert bobby pins into your hair and the foundation. Do this at the front, back, and sides, but be careful that you do not punch a hole into the cap or base.

There are two reasons for the combs and bobby pins. First, you do not want to be going north on Main Street while your hair is flying south. And this does happen! However, you can get over the loss of your dignity. The important reason is to distribute the weight of the "extra hair" to keep it from pushing and pulling on your own hair, which can weaken, break, and be damaged.

DONNING AND DOFFING

The Wig. If you have short to medium-length hair, set your hair in *dry* pincurls before putting on a wig. When you remove your wig, your hair will look neat. If you dampen or wet your pincurls, you will have a case of the "frizzies" and can damage the wig cap. Long hair can be twirled into a flat twist or wrapped around your head. All bobby pins should be slanted downward to avoid damaging the foundation.

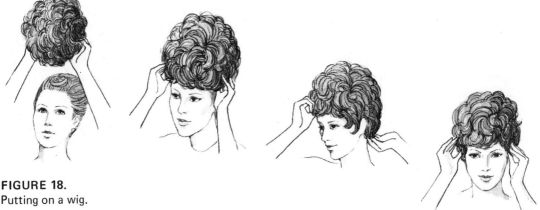

FIGURE 18.
Putting on a wig.

Study Figure 18 and follow these instructions for putting on a wig:

1. Make a base of either a flat pincurl or a crisscross of several bobby pins at the front of the head.
2. Remove the wig from the headblock by slipping your fingers under the nape of the cap and lifting forward. This will lessen the possibility of tousling the hairline.
3. Handling the wig by the temple tabs to keep from disturbing the style, tilt the wig forward over the brow. As you slide the wig—from front to back—onto your head, use one hand to glide the comb at the front of the cap into the

base of the pincurl. Use the other hand at the nape area to pull the wig down into place.

4. Carefully tuck stray strands of your hair under the wig and check to see if the temple tabs are opposite each other.

5. When your wig is positioned properly, anchor the wig to your hair with bobby pins at the nape of the neck, at the temple tabs, and at the browline.

6. With a comb, hairlift, or wig brush, touch up the edges of the hairline. If needed, spray a fine mist of hairspray.

7. To remove the wig, gently pull out the bobby pins, place your thumb under the nape of the cap, and lift forward. With your other hand, gently support the crown area. Immediately place the wig on a wig block. (To keep from stretching the wig cap, be *positive* the block is not larger than your head size.)

Hairpieces. Always style your hairpieces to compliment your individual features, and remember, business executives *strenuously* object to "after-five" coiffures during business hours. See Figures 19 and 20, and follow these suggestions for donning your hairpiece.

1. Comb and brush your own hair into the desired style. (Do not forget to make a pincurl base or a crisscross of bobby pins where the hairpiece is to be attached.)

2. Holding the foundation, position the prestyled hairpiece, slide the comb into the pincurl base, and further secure with bobby pins.

3. To position a curl or wave, permanently squeeze a hairpin close together, pull the curl or wave into the desired

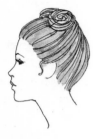 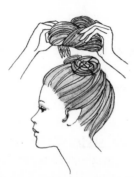 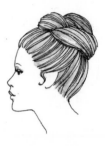

FIGURE 19.
Donning a hairpiece.

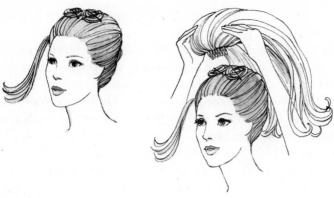

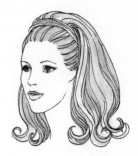

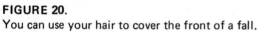

FIGURE 20.
You can use your hair to cover the front of a fall.

arrangement, and insert the hairpin as you would a bobby pin. (A bobby pin will be too obvious, and if you bend one side of the hairpin back, you will muss the style when you try to remove it.)

4. When detaching the hairpiece, gently dislodge all hairpins and bobby pins. Place your fingers under the front edge of the hairpiece and lift forward and upward. Place it on a headblock and secure it with T-pins.

If you want to cover the front fall edge with your hair, section off a portion of your front hair and gently tease before positioning the fall. After the fall has been properly placed and secured, gently brush your hair into the hair of the fall so that no "line of demarcation" shows. If you do not want to work your hair into the fall, camouflage the edge of the fall with bows, scarves, headbands, or a small switch or braid.

If your own hair needs a wiglet or cascade to give it body and height, section off the front part of your hair and tease gently. Position the hairpiece by inserting the comb into a pincurl base and anchoring with bobby pins. Then gently brush and smooth your hair back and over the hairpiece.

LITTLE THINGS MEAN A LOT

To truly enjoy your "extra hair," it should be kept in a neat coiffure, ready to wear. Naturally, each trip you make to have it cleaned and styled is costly, so you want to take the necessary precautions to keep your wigs and pieces clean and in good condition.

All human hair and synthetic wigs and hairpieces should be placed on a styrofoam block as soon as you remove them from your head. They should be gently combed or brushed to touch up the style so that they will be ready to wear. On human hair, use T-pins and rollers to hold waves and curls in place so they will not droop. Spray *lightly* with a hairspray.

If your "extra hair" is to be stored in a wig case, leave the case partially unzipped so air can circulate. If it is stored on a shelf, cover it with a light flimsy material, such as chiffon, to keep it clean.

Cleaning Synthetics. The man-made fibers lack porosity and do not need to be cleaned as often as human hair. An occasional thorough brushing will help to remove wig spray, dust, and dirt.

When the synthetic becomes soiled and needs a good cleaning, brush to remove tangles and surface dirt. Then simply submerge it in a solution of cool water and a very mild detergent (or a specially-formulated synthetic cleaner). Swish it around a bit and rinse. To clean the foundation, use a soft toothbrush or washcloth. Gently squeeze out excess water (never twist or wring the foundation), and press out moisture with a terry towel. Hang it on a clothes line in a shady spot, or place it on a block and let it dry naturally. Don't forget:

1. If you brush or comb a wet synthetic you will remove the curl.
2. You will stretch the wig cap if you place it on a wig block larger than your headsize.
3. You can damage the piece if you let it soak in the soapy solution or cleaning fluid for a prolonged period.

Cleaning Human Hair. To help stretch the budget, many women prefer to "do it themselves" instead of paying a wigologist to clean their human hair wigs and pieces. If you are a "do it yourselfer," always work in a well-ventilated room as a safety precaution.

1. Brush the wig and hairpiece thoroughly to remove snarls, spray, and dirt. Remember to start brushing at the ends and work to the top.

2. Place hair and about three ounces of a nonflammable liquid cleaner (never soap and water) in a large ceramic bowl.

3. Gently knead and dip hair in the fluid until it feels clean. If necessary, clean the edges and inside of the foundation with a soft toothbrush, cotton balls, or a washcloth. **Don't forget**: no twisting, wringing, or rubbing.

4. Remove the hair from the cleaner and gently squeeze out excess fluid. Then roll it in a terry towel to remove as much moisture as possible.

5. Place the wig or hairpiece on a plastic-covered canvas block the size of your head, and pin it in place. If you place your human hairpiece under a dryer, remember that prolonged exposure to high heat will ruin it; *it must be dried slowly with controlled low heat.* For the safest results, let it dry naturally.

Because manufacturer's instructions on using cleaning fluids can vary, it is always advantageous for you to check their directions.

YOU CAN TAKE IT WITH YOU

A woman's wig case has become more important to her as a traveling companion than her overnight case. To help keep your spare hair in good condition while traveling, you might like to try the following tips on packing:

1. If you are flying, inquire from the airline the size wig case you may carry aboard. If your wig case does not meet their specifications and you are required to check it, ask the airline personnel to place your case in a corrugated box. This will help to keep it from being damaged. (Wig cases that will slide under the seat of the plane can be purchased.)

2. If you are carrying more than one hairpiece, you can attach at least two to a headblock. For example: Place a wig or fall on the headblock as you would normally, then pin a wiglet to the face of the block.

3. Anchor your hairpiece to the headblock with T-pins, and use T-pins and rollers to hold curls and waves in place.

Wrap several long pieces of soft tissue around the hair and headblock and fasten with T-pins. This will help to keep the style from being disturbed should your wig case topple over.

4. Use strips of masking tape to anchor the headblock to the bottom of the wig case. This keeps the headblock from coming off the bottom base should the wig case turn upside down.

5. If you are caught without space for a wig case or do not have one, secure the curls and waves of your hairpiece with bobby pins, hairpins, and rollers and place the piece in a plastic bag. Blow up the bag like a balloon, and knot or tie the end. Pack it in your suitcase.

6. If you are traveling by car and do not have a wig case, insert T-pins, through the base of the styrofoam headblock, into the carpet of the car. This will keep the headblock from tumbling over.

7. When arriving at your destination, immediately restyle or touch up any tousling that may have occurred during travel so your spare hair will be ready when you need it. If you did not bring a headblock, there are certain lamps whose shades may be removed, leaving the shade base to be used as a headblock. But, *don't turn on the lamp*: The heat from the light bulb may damage your hairpiece.

IS THAT YOUR HAIR?

There will be a day—or days—when someone will say, "Is that your hair?" Look them straight in the eye, smile your sweetest smile, and say, "Yes." It is your hair . . . you bought and paid for it.

ENRICHMENT ACTIVITIES

Your Hair and Its Care

1. a. Analyze the condition and texture of your hair.
   b. Determine a daily and weekly treatment routine for your particular hair condition and texture.

2. **a.** What is the shape of your face?

    b. What facial features should you camouflage?

3. Cut out five pictures of hairstyles from magazines and newspaper ads. Paste the pictures on sheets of paper, and under each picture list the reasons why that particular style would or would not be flattering to you.

4. **a.** Write a brief description of an *informal* hairstyle that is flattering to you and your lifestyle.

    b. Write a brief description of a *formal* hairstyle that is flattering to you.

Your Spare Hair

1. Make a checklist of the features that should be considered when purchasing wigs and hairpieces.

2. **a.** List the advantages and disadvantages of human hairpieces.

    b. List the advantages and disadvantages of synthetic pieces.

    c. Which is most advantageous for you and your lifestyle? Why?

3. Write a brief description of the styles, colors, shades in spare hair that are most complimentary to you.

4. If you have wigs and/or hairpieces:

    a. Analyze the texture, body, manageability, and sheen of your spare hair.

    b. Are the strands or fibers: properly distributed＿＿＿＿ ＿＿＿＿; do they move freely in all directions ＿＿＿＿＿＿; is machine stitching uniform＿＿＿＿＿＿?

    c. Does your spare hair fit properly? What must be done for a proper fit?

    d. If your spare hair is not in good condition, list the steps and treatment needed to restore it.

5

makeup for today's look

Beauty has been a source of fascination, intrigue, and experimentation since the days of the legendary beauty, Cleopatra. Unlike Cleopatra, today's woman does not have the leisure to employ an elaborate beauty ritual. Such preoccupation with beauty often indicates an inwardness which is not becoming to a woman, no matter how lovely the outer facade.

For that glowing, healthy skin women find so desirable, it is necessary to care for the skin and body meticulously. Many products are available on the cosmetic market today, a market selling almost a billion dollars worth of cosmetics annually, but no product available will substitute for a good basic, complexion care routine.

A well-balanced diet will help maintain the proper chemical balance and assure a fresh, dewy-looking complexion: *lots* of leafy green vegetables, lean meats, eggs, cheese, and fresh fruits; a minimum of fatty or fried foods and rich desserts; and *lots* of water—at least eight tall glasses per day.

Vital as a good diet is to complexion glow, exercise, proper circulation, and sleep are equally important. Exercise works better than any facial or other stimulating cosmetic to stimulate the flow of blood to the skin. Fatigue robs the complexion of vitality and tends to accentuate tiny lines and wrinkles.

70

A VERY SPECIAL YOU

Your skin is unique to you. However, there are several general types of skin and proper ways to care for each. The products vary, but the procedure does not. The types of skin are normal, oily, dry, sensitive (one subject to allergies and blemishes), or a combination. Here are some characteristics that help distinguish the various types.

Normal: Firm, smooth texture; slight oiliness on forehead, nose, and chin. Good color with very little tendency toward blackheads or blemishes. Slight dryness around mouth and eyes. Usually possessed by those *under thirty*.

Oily: All-over oily shine. Course, heavy looking texture with flaking around nose. Enlarged pores with tendency toward blemishes, blackheads, and whiteheads. Generally poor circulation.

Dry: Parched, thirsty looking; thin, flaky texture. Noticeable lines and tiny wrinkles in eye, forehead, and above lip line. Can be very beautiful and flawless; but extreme care must be taken to combat premature aging, especially noticeable after thirty.

Sensitive: Generally the same look as dry skin, but with small, broken capillaries and traces of surface veins. This type is often susceptible to vitiligo, patches of whitened dry skin caused by loss of pigment. There are medicines available that are helpful in clearing these white spots, which are especially noticeable when skin becomes tanned.

Combination: Skin often fails to fit into one of the other four categories. The combination skin may be the blend of dry or normal skin with oily patches in the forehead, nose, and chin area. It is necessary to adjust your cleansing routine to achieve normal, well-balanced looking skin.

CLEANSING CAPERS

A basic or simplified cleansing routine is best for the involved woman in today's world. It is always fun to prepare for a special occasion by

71

taking extra time to cleanse your skin and prepare a relaxing facial, but eight o'clock in the morning and eleven o'clock in the evening are not ideal times to spend thirty minutes to an hour cleansing and stimulating the skin. *A word of caution*: Fight the impulse to pile into bed with all your makeup on simply because you are too tired tonight or will be too rushed to reapply your makeup in the morning. The pores of your skin need to breathe to be healthy. If makeup is clogging the pores, your skin will not benefit from the natural effects of a good night's sleep and the ease from tension.

The easiest and kindest beauty treatment for your skin is *sleep*. A young bride once admitted that she slept in her false eyelashes because she wanted her husband to see her at her best. True, you want to be seen at your best, but the aging effect of sleeping in false eyelashes with surgical glue affixed to the lid is inevitable. Better to cleanse the skin, use a skin freshener and a light coat of moisture cream, and apply a delicate scent before retiring. A pale lip gloss or medicated lip preparation will make you feel even more attractive and will help soften the lip line as you sleep.

Your skin must be clean—immaculately clean. Particles of dust and other pollution float in the air and settle on your skin. For this reason, you must never apply fresh makeup to a dirty face or on top of makeup that has been on for some time.

Another danger to good complexion care is the powder puff. The puff absorbs excess oil from your skin when applying either loose or compressed powder. As you use the same puff to apply another coat of powder, you are applying another coat of dirt as well. A better idea is to apply the powder with a cotton pad or ball, or a powder brush.

To help freshen makeup, carry facial tissues to blot excess oil and revitalize your makeup glow. Cotton pads moistened with astringent, skin freshener, or simply cold water applied to the face can freshen makeup and remove excess oils that tend to cause irritation.

FIVE FABULOUS STEPS TO BEAUTY

Cleansing. Removing makeup requires as much technique as applying it. See the cleansing diagram, Figure 21. Two types of products are available for your choice: (1) cream, or (2) soap, the mild types such as castile or glycerine. The makeup produced today is difficult to remove; therefore it is necessary to cleanse the face at

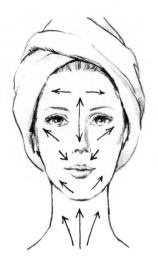

FIGURE 21.

Cleansing diagram. Work upward from the base of the neck, smoothing upward from the chin to the front of the ear. Work in the same direction until you reach the side of the nose. From the bridge of the nose, smooth lightly along the cheekbone to the temples. Use horizontal strokes from the brow to the hairline.

least twice to assure removal of *all* traces of makeup. There are foaming types of cleansers that are applied and removed with water. However, a special cream or oil is necessary to remove eye makeup. This is also true when cleansing with soap.

When applying face cream, apply it to the forehead, nose, cheeks, chin, and neck areas, working in a gentle patting motion upward and outward, taking special care in the eye area. Allow the cream to work a moment, remove it with a facial cloth or mitten made with three or four tissues wrapped securely around the fingers, working again in gentle upward-outward motion. Facial cloth is preferred to tissue because a tissue leaves microscopic bits of wood pulp residue in the pores.

If you prefer soap for cleansing, work up a good lather in the palms of the hands and gently apply the lather in a circular motion until all areas of the face and neck are covered. A word of caution about soap. Most cosmetic experts are strongly opposed to the use of soap because it has a wax base, and particles of wax are deposited in the skin causing the pores to become enlarged. They feel, also, that soap is too drying to the natural oils of the skin. Many liquid, medicated cleansing soaps that are less drying than facial soap are available, and many dermatologists recommend them.

Freshening. After cleansing, the skin should be freshened to close the pores. Because natural oils and acids have been removed from the skin, it is left vulnerable to infection and irritation. It is important to be sure all traces of cream or soap are removed. Thus you may choose (according to your skin type) a freshener, which is a mild, nondrying, nonalcoholic preparation, or an astringent, which has more drying properties, such as alcohol. For normal, dry, or sensitive skin, use a skin *freshener.* For oily or combination skin, use *astringent.* Astringent should be used on combination skin only in the oily areas: nose, forehead, and chin. When neither freshener nor astringent is available, substitute cold water or ice.

Circulating. One way to stimulate skin circulation is through exercise. You should have a vigorous exercise program. One substitute, if you do not, however, is to stand in front of an open window and run in place until you feel the blood circulate and the face tingle. Another method is to apply your cleanser, freshener, or astringent in a gentle, slapping motion until you feel the face tingle or sting a bit. Pay particular attention to the chin and neck areas. These show the tell-tale signs of aging or careless complexion care.

Facial masks are excellent to stimulate skin circulation and to refine the texture of the pores. One famous fifty-year-old beauty with a complexion of a thirty-year-old said she would give up her taxi before she gave up her weekly facial. And in New York City, that's saying a lot. This important routine should be followed weekly or more often. Ideas for facials you can prepare yourself will be discussed later in this chapter.

Lubricating. This vital step is important to the person with dry or sensitive skin. Because nature has robbed her of an abundance of oils, she must supplement with a lubricant rich in lanolin or other emollients. When exercising outdoors, especially in harsh, cold weather, a protective coating of oil is essential to the person with dry skin. Lubricants are not to be confused with moisturizers. Lubricants do as the name suggests: they add oil. Moisturizers add moisture or water. Even if you use rich creams, you should include a moisturizer, for they work hand-in-hand to maintain the proper balance of the normal skin.

All skin types require the lubricant eye cream. The eye area does not have oil glands and needs oil to keep it soft and smooth, just as all skins need moisturizers to keep skin plump and smooth-looking, not drawn and parched-looking.

Protecting. Here the elements of sun and wind come into play. Sun is one of the most aging agents to the skin. Doctors strongly advise the use of a sun screen or block when anticipating exposure to the sun for any length of time. Wind dries the skin as well and is especially harmful when combined with cold weather. The sun screen is a must for idling at the beach or swishing down the ski slopes. Sun causes blotches in the skin, sometimes called liver spots. Protect against these spots and the cancerous effects of overexposure to sun by covering your face with an attractive sun hat when outdoors, and use a long sleeve cover-up for arms and shoulders.

Freckles are made more noticeable by excessive exposure to the sun. People with freckles should habitually wear a sun screen preparation. The saying, "tan and healthy looking," is not necessarily true because tanning is actually the process of burning the pigment of the skin. Overexposure to the sun's rays is not immediately detectable except by a burning sensation followed by blisters, but the results become evident years later.

NIGHT AND DAY CARE

Normal Skin—Daytime Routine. You are the lucky one. The choice of using mild soap (glycerine or castile) or cleansing cream is yours. You might want to use the cleansing cream first and follow it with a mild soap sudsing.

If you use cream, apply it to the face and neck area, using a gentle upward and outward motion with the tips of the fingers, taking special care not to tug or pull. Gently apply eye makeup remover to the eye area. Allow both creams to work a few minutes. Remove makeup with a facial cloth, again working in an upward-outward motion. More harm is done by removing makeup improperly than by failing to remove makeup at all.

Follow cleansing with freshening. Dip cotton balls or pads in cold water, squeeze out the excess, and then moisten with freshener. Gently apply it to all areas of the face and neck to assure removal of all excess cream or traces of soap.

Dot moisturizer cream or lotion onto forehead, below the brow line, cheek, chin, and on both sides of the neck. Smooth in the moisturizer with the tips of the fingers. Allow one minute for your skin to absorb the moisturizer, and remove the excess with a cotton ball, pad, or tissue. Contrary to popular belief, moisturizer *will not* make the skin oilier. The skin will absorb only the amount of moisture needed to maintain water balance. Consider this routine as an artist preparing a canvas—you are the artist and are now ready to paint (makeup) the picture (your face).

Normal Skin—Nighttime Routine. The nighttime routine is the same as the daytime routine with the exception of applying makeup. You will want to apply a thin coat of night cream or oil-base lubricating cream after the moisturizer. As in all makeup procedures, apply gently, patting it in an upward-outward motion. Dot a thin coat of eye cream on the eye area because this is where the "crow's feet" or telltale lines begin to form first. The old adage, "an ounce of prevention is worth a pound of cure," certainly applies. The cost of eye cream may seem excessive, but you use only a tiny bit for each application, and the supply will last for months. The same is true of moisturizers. Normal skin needs a facial each week to maintain that healthy, well-balanced texture.

Oily Skin—Daytime Routine. The oily skin, characterized by its all-over shine and coarse texture, must be cleansed even more thoroughly and frequently than the normal skin, at least twice a day when possible. Soap is excellent for oily skin. Castile or glycerine soap is applied by circulating the lather to the forehead, nose, cheek, chin, and neck areas in an upward-outward motion to remove oil and dirt deposits. Cleansing granules are helpful to refine the texture of the oily skin.

If you prefer a cleansing cream, use only formulas developed for oily skin. Apply two coats to the face and neck area, smoothing it in carefully and working upward and outward to prevent pulling. Apply eye makeup remover to the eye area. Give both creams a few minutes to penetrate the makeup. Remove the makeup with a facial cloth or mitten of tissue (three or four tissues wrapped around the fingers and secured with the thumb).

Briskly pat astringent pads on all areas of the face and neck to assure the complete removal of all traces of makeup and to close and tighten pores.

You alone will have to determine whether you wear a light film of moisturizer under your makeup during the day. Moisturizer helps in smoothing makeup on more evenly, but some oily skins fairly "drip" oil; if you have this type of skin, you may choose not to add a moisturizer for daytime.

Oily skin benefits from frequent facials, which help decrease oil pockets, stimulate circulation, and refine the pore texture. The complexion brush is beneficial to oily skin in helping to increase circulation and in removing dirt from clogged pores. Special soaps such as tar soap or tincture of green soap may be recommended by your dermatologist if your skin problems are acute.

Oily Skin—Nighttime Routine. The nighttime routine is the same as the daytime routine except that you must apply eye cream to the eye area and may choose to apply a medicated drying cream to the face. Calamine lotion is helpful for clearing up minor surface blemishes. For extreme skin problems, consult a dermatologist. Acne and permanent scarring may easily be avoided if the skin is treated in time. See Guide 1 for information on acne control.

GUIDE 1

Acne Control

1.   Acne is a disease aggravated by bacteria and hormonal imbalance during adolescence.

2.   Wash your face daily with the finger tips as often as needed.

3.   Shampoo your hair every one to four days as necessary to keep your scalp clean; leave the shampoo on for five full minutes before rinsing.

4.   To look neat, use cosmetics as little as possible. Avoid pancake makeup and heavy powders. Many good, hypoallergenic cosmetics are available and designed especially for sensitive skin.

5.   Keep your hair as short as is becoming to your face type. This makes shampooing less time-consuming.

6.   Excessive emotional stress can cause considerable aggravation of skin problems. Eight hours of sleep a night is as necessary as outdoor exercise and drinking lots of water.

7.   Avoid picking pimples—keep your hands from your face.

8.   Avoid chocolate, nuts, cola, milk and milk products, citrus fruits, fatty foods, shell fish (iodine is bad for acne), spinach, and spicy foods, being especially careful if one food type causes noticeable skin flareups for you.

9.   Apply local medication to dry up active pimples by reducing excessive oil and skin debris. Remember: Excessive or abrasive cleaning will irritate the skin.

10.   Your acne cannot be cured, but it can be controlled. Some cases are more difficult to control than others. See a dermatologist to help avoid emotional problems resulting from skin problems and a permanent scarring of your face and personality. Start your skin care and acne control program *today*!

11.   If your face becomes scarred with acne, you may have your

dermatologist clear these scars with dermabrasion, or with chemosurgery. Chemosurgery and dermabrasion noticeably improve skin texture and are not particularly painful, considering the remarkable results achieved.

Dry Skin—Daytime Routine. Dry skin can be the most beautiful of all skins because of the fine, porcelain-like texture. Although dry skin is more susceptible to fine lines and wrinkles than normal or oily skin, there are fewer problems with blackheads and other blemishes.

The key to maintaining this beautiful skin is careful cleansing and moisturizing. Generously apply a rich cleansing cream to the entire face and neck area. With gentle motions, remove the cream with a facial cloth or tissue mitten in an upward-outward motion. Take special care in applying and removing eye makeup remover cream. The eye area is very delicate and will stretch and wrinkle if rubbed too harshly.

Apply a skin freshener in a gentle, patting motion to the forehead, nose, cheek, chin, and neck area. Faithfully apply a moisturizer or protective lotion to the entire face and neck area after cleansing and freshening.

Winter climate and harsh winds are harmful to dry skin. You may need to use a light lubricating cream under your makeup if your skin is especially dry or if you are exercising outdoors for any length of time.

A mild, non-irritating facial designed for dry skin will help the woman with dry skin retain her fine pores. Every seven to ten days is often enough for your facials. Your facial is for circulatory purposes rather than for skin refinement.

Dry Skin—Nighttime Routine. The woman with dry skin must clean her face religiously each evening because makeup will dry even more of the precious oils in the skin when left on overnight. After cleansing carefully with a rich cleansing cream, freshen the face with cotton pads dipped in skin freshener and add a rich night cream to pamper your skin. Gently apply eye cream to the eye area to prevent formation of crow's feet.

Sensitive Skin—Day-Night Routine. The sensitive skin must be treated the same as dry skin. However, particular care must be taken in selecting the proper skin care products and cosmetics. If your skin has tiny rashes or other irritations, it may be necessary to use a special skin cream, lotion, or antibiotic product in your nighttime routine. Use cleansing and stimulating products that are hypoallergenic and designed especially for sensitive skin. Be dedicated to a thorough skin care routine.

Combination Skin—Day-Night Routine. The combination skin, because of its dual nature, can be treated with alternating cream and soap cleansings. It is suggested that the morning cleansing be a *soap* and water application, followed by skin *freshener* and a moisturizer.

The nighttime routine could include a cleansing cream application and removal followed by astringent for those troublesome oily spots—forehead, nose, and chin line. Lightly apply a moisturizer, blotting off all the excess, and pat on eye cream to the delicate eye area.

THAT FACE—THAT FABULOUS FACIAL

Facials are fun. They serve two purposes. One is to increase circulation and the other is to ease tension lines and other aging signs. Many facial products are available, from cucumber concoctions to watermelon wraps, but the facials to be discussed in this section are those you can prepare at home. They are pure products and fun to work with, though sometimes a bit messy! The kind of facial you use is determined by the main ingredient of the facial, that is, salt, cornmeal, and so forth. Apply the facial above the browline and below the eye socket bone.

Honey Facial. Always start with a thoroughly cleaned face. Cleanse the face gently and massage it to increase circulation. Remove the cream and gently pat on honey around the eyes. Press your fingers against your face and pull them away quickly, using the stickiness of the honey to stimulate circulation. Continue this procedure for three minutes. Steam the face with a warm, damp towel, removing the excess honey. Follow this with a towel dipped in ice water. Pat on skin freshener or astringent.

Dry Skin Facial. Cleanse the face with cream. Remove the cream carefully. Use a second application of cream and massage it into the skin. Apply a hot, damp towel and gently press it against the skin. Follow this with a generous application of skin oil, removing the excess oil with a soft cloth. Immediately apply a second hot towel for one minute. Complete the facial by patting on a skin freshener. Either baby oil or olive oil (if you can stand the smell) may be used.

Oily Skin—Epsom Salt Facial. The epsom salt facial helps you relax and it stimulates your circulation. Clean the face thoroughly. Place two bowls in front of you, with hot water in one and cold water with ice cubes in the other. Using two tablespoons of epsom salt to one pint water, add the salt to each bowl and stir until it is dissolved. Wring a towel in the hot water solution and hold it against your face and neck. Apply the towel with hot solution five times. Soak the towel in the cold water solution and apply it to your face and neck ten times. Complete the treatment with a light coat of moisture cream or lotion.

Cornmeal Mask. Clean the skin thoroughly. Mix a quarter cup of yellow cornmeal and enough buttermilk to make a thin, though not runny, paste. Spread it on a cheesecloth mask or directly onto skin. Moisten the mask with extra buttermilk and let it dry about fifteen minutes. Remove it from the face with warm water. Apply a skin freshener. This mask acts as a mild facial bleach. To make buttermilk, stir a tablespoon of lemon juice or vinegar into a cup of sweet milk.

Yeast Facial. Clean the face thoroughly. Mix half a yeast cake with enough milk or water to make a smooth paste. Smooth it onto the face and leave it for fifteen minutes. Remove it with warm water. Apply a skin freshener or astringent.

Salt Facial. The salt facial is especially good for blackhead-prone areas. Clean the skin gently but thoroughly. Place one tablespoon of cleansing cream in the palm of your hand and sprinkle it generously with salt until it feels grainy. Apply it in a gentle, circular motion to blackhead areas. Leave it on your skin for five minutes. If it starts to burn slightly, remove it immediately. This treatment is also effective when applied to blemishes on the back.

MAKEUP—THE ARTIST AT WORK

Just as the artist prepares his canvas before creating a masterpiece, you use the techniques you have learned for preparing your canvas, your face, for an experience in makeup artistry. Painting a prettier you is our goal—lightly, if you please.

Begin by assembling your tools, brushes of all sorts. Makeup brushes may be purchased at the cosmetic counter; but art brushes in all widths, textures, and sizes are available at art or office-supply houses, often at substantial savings.

Your paints will be your makeup base or foundation, powder, eye shadow, and lipstick. Now let us journey into the artistry of makeup. First, study the twenty steps to applying makeup listed in Guide 2.

GUIDE 2

Steps To Follow in Applying Makeup

1. Splash the face with cold water.
2. Wring a cotton pad out in cold water. Saturate it with freshener if your skin is normal or dry, or with astringent if your skin is oily. Pat it over your face and neck, using upward motions.
3. Apply a wrinkle lotion around the eye area and other places where it is needed.
4. Apply a moisturizer. Let it set for a few minutes.
5. Cover the dark area under your eyes with a product designed for this purpose. Blend it with a small brush.
6. Stroke foundation over the face, and blend it carefully down into the neck area.
7. Use a tiny brush and apply white highlights (use a cream type) under the outer eyebrow area.
8. Stroke a line of taupe cream eye shadow across the bone above your eye.
9. Dot a small amount of cream rouge on the cheek bones, chin, and hairline. Blend it in. (You can use lipstick if it is a creamy type.) Pinkish colors are best.
10. Using a *sponge* powder puff, press and smooth a small amount of light, transparent powder over your face and neck. Smooth it firmly down the side of your face where facial hair has a tendency to grow more thickly.
11. Brush the eyebrows down. Fill in along the top of the brow line with short, feathery strokes; then brush the brows up and into shape. There will be no telltale lines at the lower edge of the brow!
12. Optional: A tiny bit of eyebrow pencil may be dotted from the middle to the outer corner underneath the eye. Blend them so that the dots run together.

13.   Using a light, powdered eye shadow and small brush strokes, color along the top of the lid, into the corner, and with a thin, soft line, just under the lower lashes (more at night). Blue is good on almost every complexion and blends with most clothing colors. Avoid weird colors of eye shadows.

14.   Apply false lashes at this point if you choose to wear them.

15.   Apply a thin streak of eyeliner across the top of the eye, just at the roots of the lashes. Use cake eyeliner and a tiny sable brush or one of the new wands created for this purpose. Do not use eyebrow pencil as it stretches the eyelid.

16.   Apply mascara to the bottom lashes and, if you have not used false lashes, to the top ones. Even if you are using extra lashes, you may use just a little mascara on them.

17.   With a brush, make a *tiny* dot of white highlight cream at the outer corner and at the inner corner of eyes. Blend them in.

18.   Brush blusher lightly onto the cheekbones, hairline, and chin.

19.   Outline the lip line with a lipbrush, lip pencil, or brown eyebrow pencil. Fill it in with medium color—neither a red red that dates you, nor the pale color, whose deathly look also dates you.

20.   Finally, pat the face and neck with moist hands. Or you may again saturate a cotton pad in cold water, wring it out, and pat it over your face. This will *set* your makeup and help keep it looking fresh for hours.

The Artist Chooses Her Subject. Don't let the title mislead you. Have you ever watched an artist work? Everyone is an artist in one way or another. Makeup can be a very pleasing form of artistic expression. You have learned that preparing your skin is the first step. Once the skin is meticulously groomed you are ready to begin the sketch.

The shape you are working with will be the shape of your face. Do you know what shape your face is? There are several ways to help you decide. One is to place your face close to the mirror, with your nose touching it, and with a bit of cream trace the outline of your face on the mirror. This may not be exact, but it will be a guide. Another way is to visit a cosmetic counter and let a makeup expert analyze your face and skin. This is fun, and you may want to try several experts to be sure their analyses agree.

The Sensuous Seven—Facial Shapes, of Course—Upon determining your facial structure, you may use the following descriptions as a guide in applying makeup properly to enhance your most pleasing features. (See Figures 22 through 28 for illustration of these techniques.) National surveys conducted by CPI show that men notice the eye before any other facial feature. Therefore, illustrations depicting eye makeup will also be shown.

First, your face!

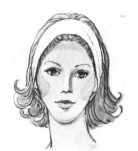

Diamond: This face has a narrow forehead and narrow chin and is often a tiny face as well. Taupes or darker foundation should be applied under the chin area to shorten and soften the pointed look. Use soft blush in the forehead area to soften the triangular shape. Rouge should be well-placed below the eye and extending to the outer corner of eye.

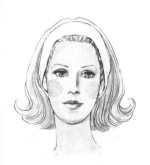

Rectangle: The rectangular face has a long, squared shape. Contour the area under the chin and jaw line with taupe or darker foundation to slim its squareness. Rouge starts at the outer edge of the iris of the eye, extending almost to the top of the ear line, and tapers out at the ear lobe.

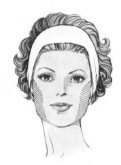

Square: The square face is a short face. You must work to create the illusion of length. Soften the jowls with shadow. Avoid hairstyles that fall at the chin line and further emphasize the face's squareness. Rouge must be placed high on the cheek bones and confined to a small area of the upper face. Do not shorten the length of your face by extending color below the earlobe.

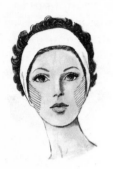

Circle: The round face needs height to create an elongated look. Apply blush in the area underneath the cheek line. Draw the face in (imitate the fish look). Apply a blush where the hollows appear. This will cut the effect of roundness. Use a slightly darker base on the lower half of the face to create a sloping effect. Carefully feather in lines of foundation tones from the upper to the lower face.

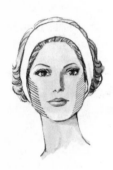

Pear: The narrowness in the temple area is best filled in with hair, but another alternative is to apply blush to the forehead to reduce the angular shape. The fullness in lower part of the cheek can be contoured by shadowing the jawline. Taupe or darker foundation works nicely to create these shadows.

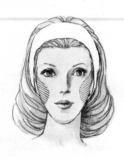

Heart: This is another rather small facial type. The fullness in the temple area can be minimized by keeping hair close to the temples, and by placing the rouge in a triangular shape just below the eye, extending it downward almost an inch and outward an inch to the corner of the eye. The chin tends to come to a point, so soften the angle by using a lighter base or shadow to create the illusion of roundness.

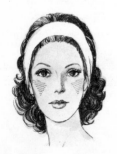

Oval: Yours is the shape others are striving to achieve. You may experiment with many types of makeup shading for the effect you *choose* to create. A balanced blush or rouge line applied with fullest part in line with the top and bottom of the ear and triangle coming to a point at the cheekbone is most flattering.

Tone on Tone. The predominant color of your skin will fall within the tones ranging from yellow, pink, and blue-white to black. Texture of pores sometimes causes a focusing of the eye on your skin with added intensity. For example, those skins severely affected by acne and scarring will tend to develop a reddish cast or glow.

It is important to select a foundation color that complements your natural color. Foundation can be used to diminish or correct certain obvious skin tones. The foundation should be at least one or two shades darker than the skin. If your skin is a bit too yellow, or sallow, a slightly peachy tone base will brighten the dull look. If your skin is too red, a beige tone base can minimize the redness and add a softness to the face.

The black woman is the lucky one, for the line of cosmetics for her is absolutely unique. It employs the whole spectrum of colors from pale coppery tones to the rich mahogany shades. The shine is lovely, and the eye makeup so soft and frosted it emphasizes the eye dramatically. Blush and other beauty care products available for her are fantastic.

The blue-white skin tone, usually possessed by brunettes and redheads, needs a soft, peach-cream tone to balance the porcelain white.

The Color Chart, Table 1, is a complete guide to help a woman choose a makeup base or foundation right for her.

One important factor that enters into selecting the right foundation color is your body's *chemical* balance. What may appear to be just the right shade base for you when you apply it may later turn a different color. It is wise to test a base on the throat area. If the base blends the throat to the facial tone, you will never have a telltale line. Allow the base to set for several minutes. Then reapply the same base to a nearby area on the throat and judge whether or not the color has changed significantly. If not, buy it!

CHOOSING YOUR ART FORM

Just as the artist chooses the type color media he is to work with—oil, acrylic, water color, charcoal, or pen and ink—you must choose the kind of foundation you wish to work with—cream, lotion, stick, cake, or gel. The effect you wish to create will help you decide which kind to use.

The light cream or lotion form will give a filmy, natural look.

TABLE 1

Color chart

Skin	Foundation	Powder	Lipstick	Cheek Rouge	Hair
Blonde, light skin	Natural (very light)	Lightweight non-coloring	Light orange-red	Light orange-red	Light blonde
Blonde, medium skin	Faintly pink	Lightweight non-coloring	Pale strawberry	Pale strawberry	Medium blonde
Blonde, sallow skin	A light blue-red	Lightweight non-coloring	Light blue-red	Light blue-red	Dark blonde
Blonde, reddish skin	A peach buff	Lightweight non-coloring	True pepper red	True pepper red	Ash blonde
Blonde, dark skin	A warm copper	Lightweight non-coloring	Medium blue-red	Medium blue-red	Reddish blonde
Red head, light skin	A faintly pink or light blue-red	Lightweight non-coloring	Pale strawberry	Pale strawberry	Strawberry blonde
Red head, medium skin	A pale peach buff	Lightweight non-coloring	True pepper red	True pepper red	Copper blonde
Red head, sallow skin	A warm rose glow	Lightweight non-coloring	Medium blue-red	Medium blue-red	Medium red
Red head, reddish skin	A peach buff	Lightweight non-coloring	Medium blue-red or pale strawberry	Medium blue-red or pale strawberry	Light auburn
Red head, dark skin	A warm copper	Lightweight non-coloring	True pepper red	True pepper red	Light brown
Brunette, light skin	Faintly pink or a light blue-red	Lightweight non-coloring	Medium blue-red	Medium blue-red	Medium brown
Brunette, medium skin	A pale peach buff	Lightweight non-coloring	Medium blue-red or a pink-red	Medium blue-red or a pink-red	Dark brown
Brunette, sallow skin	A warm rose glow	Lightweight non-coloring	Medium blue-red	Medium blue-red	Henna brown
Brunette, reddish skin	A peach buff	Lightweight non-coloring	Medium blue-red or a pink-red	Medium blue-red or a pink-red	Black
Brunette, dark skin	A warm copper	Lightweight non-coloring	Deep blue-red	Deep blue-red	Dark gray
Gray, light skin	Light blue-red	Lightweight non-coloring	Light blue-red	Light blue-red	Medium gray
Gray, medium skin	Faintly pink or a warm rose glow	Lightweight non-coloring	A light blue-red	A light blue-red	Light gray
Gray, dark skin	A peach buff	Lightweight non-coloring	A pink-red	A pink-red	White

Note:—A peach buff foundation is particularly good for summer-to-winter transition on any type, and is flattering to ruddy, sallow, or freckled skin.

Source: *Encyclopedia Americana*, Vol. 18, 1958, p.157

The skin tone will shine through. The cake or stick form will cover more thoroughly and provide a matte look. Some people prefer a matte look with frosty blush and eye shadow for night wear and a more natural soft shadow for day and sportwear. If you are blessed with a light trace of freckles, you may want to choose a base to blend the freckles in. Do not try to cover them completely. This will create a mask-like look. Freckles are the beauty mark of many beautiful women.

If your skin is troubled with acne or other blemish problems, choose a medicated or hypoallergenic base. The base often causes more problems to the sensitive skin than any other cosmetic product.

Birthmarks cannot be covered completely, but they can be blended in with proper makeup application to appear less noticeable. The cake or stick-form base will give best results for blending in these discolorations. Gel foundation is merely a blush and does little to cover any traces of discoloration, freckles, or tiny wrinkles. It is especially useful in giving a well-tanned face that beautiful bronze glow.

The actual method of applying foundation is simple. To a clean face, apply the foundation in dots on the forehead, nose, eye, chin, cheek, and throat area. In light, feathery strokes, using an upward-outward motion, work in the foundation to completely and smoothly cover all the facial areas, including the eye. Special care must be taken in applying makeup to the eye area to prevent stretching and wrinkling, as illustrated in Figure 29.

Camouflage. You may apply a product to lighten dark circles under the eyes before you put on foundation. Special color sticks, creams, or a lighter foundation shade will accomplish this. When

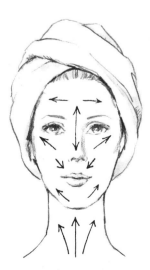

FIGURE 29.
Follow the arrows in this illustration when you apply makeup. Use the fingertips and light, feathery strokes to prevent tugging.

working to hide circles or tiny wrinkles in the eye area, include a bit of protective medicine such as a special eye cream. Eye cream keeps the eye area from drying and allows smoother application of makeup. Color sticks may be used effectively to lighten tiny smile wrinkles and to hide blemishes or small areas of discoloration on the face. The best results are acquired if the camouflaging is done before the makeup base is applied.

BLUSHING BEAUTY

A great beauty product that is constantly being manufactured in new forms is the blush. Previously, only rouge in cake or cream forms was available for the women who wanted to recapture that youthful blush. Blush is easier and quicker to apply than rouge.

The woman whose skin is dry may want to use a cream rouge, which is less desiccating. Blush can give the face an all-over rosy glow, because it can be applied to give just a hint of color. Effective results in contouring can be achieved with blush, but these results are not long-lasting.

Foundation produces a pleasing effect when one uses darker shades to create shadows and reduce fullness, or lighter shades to lighten and broaden a narrow forehead or pointed chin. The effect will last until your makeup is removed.

Blush may be chosen to complement your natural skin tone or to create a dramatic effect by complementing the outfit you wear. Apply blush sparingly. Cream blush is applied over the foundation *before* powdering and powder blush is applied *after* powdering.

COLOR FOR THE FACE

Rouge, the most popular form of color for years, has the advantage of being available in many forms and gives longer-lasting color than blush. You may choose cake, cream, liquid, or gel.

The liquid and gel go on smoothly and can be smoothed into the desired effect before the color sets. Liquid or gel is applied to the foundation *before* powder is applied. Cake or cream rouge may be applied *after* powder is used. Rouge is a bit more difficult than blush to work with because the color is more intense.

Extreme caution should be taken to avoid the "painted lady" result regardless of what the latest fashion fad suggests. As the artist paints in soft, sparing strokes, you must employ his techniques in applying your makeup. Study rouge camouflage tricks in Figures 30 and 31.

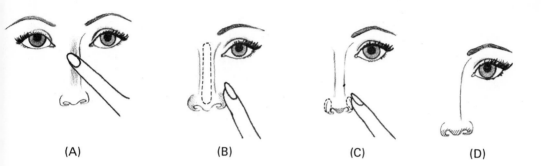

(A)   (B)   (C)   (D)

FIGURE 30.

(A) The hooked nose. Apply a darker shade of foundation over the area of nose that is hooked. (B) The broad nose. Apply a lighter shade of foundation down the center of the nose and a darker foundation to subdue flared nostrils. (C) The thin nose. Create width with lighter foundation on the nostrils, and shorten the length with darker foundation on the tip of the nose. (D) The long nose. Shorten a long nose by applying a darker shade under the tip and around the edges of the nostrils.

FIGURE 31.

(A) To make your eyes appear wider, dab a bit of rouge over the brows and on the nose tip, blending it upward and outward. (B) To raise a low brow and to highlight and warm the color of your cheeks, use a frosted white blusher just above the eyebrows out to the hairline, and blend liquid or cream rouge (pink or tawny) at the angles shown. (C) For hair worn off the face and behind the ears, put white frosting on the eartops and blend colored rouge on the bridge of your nose, outward over the brows. (D) For the round, flat face, apply rouge upward and outward on the forehead and chin and upward on the nose. Use white frosting under the brow. (E) Reduce the contrast between a pale face and a tan body with a tawny blusher.

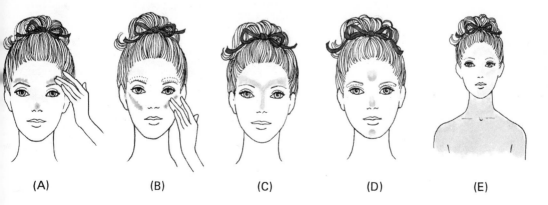

(A)   (B)   (C)   (D)   (E)

POWDER—THE FINISHING TOUCH

Women often remark that they like a natural glow. So why use powder? The chief properties of powder are its ability to set makeup for longer-lasting enjoyment and the softening, smoothing effect it gives to edges of makeup lines around rouge, cream eye shadow, and the lips.

Proper finish in applying powder results from the use of the correct tools such as a powder brush or large art brush, cotton pads or balls, sponge puffs, or traditional powder puffs. The powder brush is the preferred applicator because the powder can be applied lightly and stroked away gently to produce a delicate effect. The cotton balls or pads have the advantage of being disposable and therefore do not return dirt and oils to the skin as the powder puff does. Each time the puff is used, oils are absorbed from the skin, only to be returned with the next application of powder. Many people enjoy the dewy look the sponge puff gives the finished face. The sponge puff can easily be washed after each use.

Apply a generous amount of translucent powder to the forehead, nose, cheeks, eyes, chin, lips, and jaw line. Translucent powder is suggested because you do not want to *cover* or *destroy* the color achieved with your other makeup. Smooth lightly until powder is blended in, taking care to brush downward so that the facial hair is smooth. When the desired look has been obtained, gently press a damp cloth or cotton ball over the entire face and neck to remove excess powder and to add a soft, moist glow.

THE EYE—A MIRROR OF THE SOUL

Men admit that the look of a woman's eye immediately draws their attention. It can be a suggestive look or suggestive makeup, but

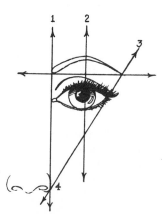

FIGURE 32.
Follow this illustration to create the illusion of a perfect eye. (1) The brow line begins. (2) The arch forms here. (3) The brow line ends. (4) Nostril of the nose.

whichever the reason, important results can be achieved by carefully and artistically applied eye makeup. First take a careful look at the diagram of the perfect eye shown in Figure 32.

Brow Shaping. As you study this diagram, take the eye test. Use a pencil as suggested in Figure 32 and check to see if your brow line falls within these limits. The next point to check is the arch line. Do you have a graceful curve with the arch coming in line with the pupil or slightly to the outside of the pupil?

Fashion dictates the change in brow line each season as it does the fashion in dress, but care must be employed in changing the line. The thin, arched line of the twenties is not flattering to most facial features, no matter what magazines suggest.

When you have determined the brow line and what must be done to improve the shape, heed a word of caution. Do not immediately pick up a pair of tweezers and go to work. Experiment with an eyebrow pencil. Draw a line you consider pleasing over or within your natural brow and study the appearance awhile. Remove that line and try another shape. It is much easier to form a line with a pencil, before removing the hairs, than it is to pencil in hairs where you have plucked them.

Then begin to create the perfect line by carefully removing the hairs a few at a time from the underside of the brow. If care is not exercised, you may end up looking like the most surprised woman in

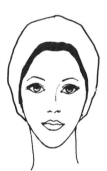

FIGURE 33.
If your face is diamond-shaped, you can make your forehead seem broader by slightly shortening the brow line.

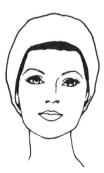

FIGURE 34.
If your face is square-shaped, you can make the forehead seem narrower by lengthening the brow line slightly to make the eyes appear more close-set.

your class or office. Apply alcohol to the brow line before and after pulling the hair to prevent infection.

Use tight tweezers, not the ones that you use to repair your jewelry, tighten a screw, or perform other household repair jobs. There are several types of tweezers such as blunt edge, pointed edge, angle edge, rounded edge, and scissor type. Select the style that is easiest for you to handle.

Study Figures 33 and 34 to learn techniques to make your forehead seem broader if your face is diamond-shaped or narrower if your face is rectangular or square-shaped. Altering your brow line will make eyes appear close-set or wider apart. These changes in the brow line are slight, not drastic. Brushing the brow regularly is necessary for a neat curving line. A little petroleum jelly or baby oil worked into the brow at bedtime, followed by a gentle brushing with a brow brush or soft toothbrush, will help unruly brows relax and will stimulate growth of sluggish brows.

Brow Coloring. To create the brow line desired, pencil in tiny, short strokes using a sharp charcoal, taupe, or navy/black pencil. If you have very little color in your brow or very little natural hair, you may choose to have your brows colored regularly. This is a simple step if you have it done by a *professional.*

It is possible for a person to color the brows and lashes herself, but people are often highly allergic to the dyes used and the results may be dangerous. An uncomfortable itching, redness, rash, or, in some instances, loss of hair may occur. A dye test *must* be made before experimenting with any hair dye or color. Remember, you do not want the brow line to jump out at you in comic movie fashion. Its color should be soft to blend in with the hair color and facial tone.

Blondes, natural and others, often need to tone down the color of their brows by working in a bit of facial powder and brushing them well. This keeps the colors in harmony.

Eyebrow Pencil. Brow pencils come in many forms, from the best-known pencil type, which is sharpened with a pencil sharpener, to slim-line pencils encased in metal, to brush-on powders. More important than the type of brow pencil you choose is the fact that you keep the point very sharp, apply the makeup in tiny, feathery strokes, and keep the shape and size of both brows uniform. *Never draw on a line.* Brush the brow lightly with a brow brush or toothbrush so that the pencil strokes blend in well with the natural hairs. If the effect is still a bit unnatural, fluff on a bit of blush or face powder to achieve the pleasing natural effect.

Subtle Shadows. Eye color is meant to enhance the natural color and not to overwhelm. A woman with vibrant blue eyes should use soft blue shadow to emphasize the color of the eye. A dark, bright blue shadow would merely drain the color from the eye.

One simple rule to remember is that light tones highlight and emphasize prominent or attractive features. To deemphasize or camouflage facial flaws, use dark tones such as taupes, mauves, and charcoals. The dark colors produce shadows and help to contour features.

Blue eyes are flattered by the use of soft blues, smoky blues, light grays, and any other color you choose to complement a costume or create a special effect.

Green eyes are naturally complemented by the use of greens, soft moss or leaf, taupes, lilac, or mauve.

Brown eyes look loveliest with taupes, greens, and soft dusky blues. Here again, color carefully applied to the lid to complement a costume is recommended.

One pleasing eye effect is produced by applying shadow directly above the lash line, feathering it out at the corner of the eye. Apply taupe, mauve, or charcoal in the crease, blending it carefully with the color line. Finish under the brow line with lightly frosted white shadow, powder, or cream if you choose to complete the look. Perhaps you would like to work a bit of colored shadow just below the lower lash to complete the look.

At this point you will want to be sure all circles or discolorations in the lower eye area have been hidden. Perhaps you didn't notice a shadow before applying the eye makeup, but one has appeared since. Use light base makeup, cream shadow stick in natural skin tones, or pale white eye cream to erase these shadows.

Use the artist's brush and touch to be sure all areas of eye color are blended in perfectly. You do not want obvious lines denoting various color applications. It takes practice, so don't be discouraged if your first few attempts produce less than expected results.

Flattering Fringe. Lucky the woman who has a thick fringe of lashes that curve gracefully and frame her eye. The other ninety-nine percent of us just have to work a bit harder to achieve this effect. Thank heavens for the marvelous mascara products available at your favorite cosmetic counter or drugstore. With a little bit of help from my friend, as the saying goes, you can add length and fullness to your lashes.

Careful attention must be paid to applying the mascara to the entire length of the lash and to brushing afterwards to separate the lashes and make them appear heavier. The powder applied to your lashes when you are powdering your face will also make the lashes appear thicker.

The choice of mascara is yours. Available are roll-on (the simplest type to apply and to carry in your purse), cake, and liquid types. Colors range from black to white. For special effect or a coordinated eye, you may want to try navy blue mascara with coordinating tones of blue for the shadow from the lashes to the brow line.

Redheads, blondes, and others with very light lashes may enjoy the effect of using taupe or chocolate brown mascara. Charcoal black gives a softer effect for brunettes and others with dark lashes, and black is alluring for the very dark, full lashes.

Care is to be taken in removing tiny dots of mascara that collect in the corners of the eye and where the fringe meets the eye. Mascara may be applied to the lower lash if the mascara is given time to dry completely. The lash is then brushed to distribute extra particles of mascara, and every trace of excess mascara is removed from the lower eye area. If your eyes are allergic and tend to tear easily, it is best to omit the makeup from the lower lash. Eye makeup for the woman who has allergic or sensitive eyes is available in many leading cosmetic lines.

To finish the fringe with a graceful curve, curl the lash with an eyelash curler. Curl the lashes carefully when the mascara is dry and lashes have been brushed. After curling, you may want to apply another light coat of mascara to the *tips* of the lashes for a definite emphasis.

In caring for your eyelash curler, be sure the rubber liner is kept solid, not ridged or cut. Otherwise, the curler will tend to pull and break the lashes. If you curl your lashes daily or more often, take time at night to work in a bit of baby oil or eye cream and brush the lashes carefully to keep them strong, healthy, and pliable.

Eye Liner. Eye liner serves a definite purpose when applying fake lashes, but it has lost its importance as a basic step in eye makeup today. The Cleopatra line, which was heavy, winged, and unnatural looking, may be appropriate for the stage or screen, but it is not the look American businessmen have endorsed so strongly and frequently. One common complaint is about heavy eye makeup, especially eye liner, combined with thick, fake lashes and contact lenses. The combination produces an irritating effect not only to the wearer but also to her coworkers who must watch her constantly batting her eyes because of eye fatigue or eye irritations.

When eye liner is used, apply the line close to the lash in a very thin, smooth manner. Use charcoal, taupe, or blue/black liner, never harsh black. Black creates an aging, unnatural effect. A thick line can make the eye appear smaller. The larger the eye appears, the more attractive it is.

Frankly Fake. Fake eyelashes can improve the eyes' appearance when they are properly applied. This technique, like most makeup techniques, takes time and practice. Carefully study Figures 35a through 35d.

A good false lash to start experimenting with is the demi-lash. This is applied to the outer two-thirds of the eye. It is easier to work with because glue that collects in the inner corner of the eyes during

FIGURE 35.
(A) If your fake lashes are too long for your eye, snip off excess hairs with small, sharp manicure scissors and put a drop of colorless nail polish on the cut end to prevent additional hairs from dropping off. (B) Feather the ends of your fake lashes for a soft, natural effect. Place them on a flat surface and gently scrape the tips with a razor blade or manicure scissors held at an angle. Taper them by snipping each hair separately, and match both strips. (C) To apply adhesive, put a drop of surgical glue on the side of a round, wooden toothpick. Run the lash base over this spot. (D) Use tweezers to put on your lashes; tip the head at an angle, and apply the lashes as close to the roots as possible. Press down with your fingers at the center point and work toward the corners. Use the flat end of an orange stick to gently secure the lashes. Place a finger on the eyelid to gently roll the skin over the lash base, and release it.

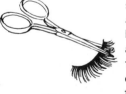
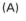

(A)

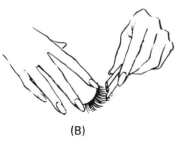

(B)

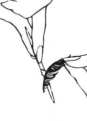
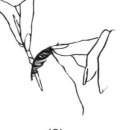

(C)

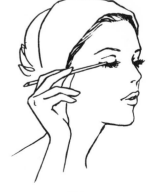

(D)

application of full lashes produces a tearing and fluttering reaction, making application of lashes difficult.

First, flex the lash to conform to the contour of the eye. Apply *surgical* glue to the base of the lash in a thin strip, using a straight pin, hair pin, or toothpick.

Allow the glue to become tacky (about thirty or forty seconds), and with a tweezer or lash applicator, apply the fake lash to the natural lash line. To do this more easily, get your face close to the mirror, tilt your chin, look down into the mirror, and open your mouth. Opening the mouth helps to steady the eye.

Now, apply the lash as close as possible to the lash line. Pat it in place with a hair pin, tweezers, or tip of a makeup brush.

The final step is to gently and carefully squeeze the fake lash and natural lash together so they adhere securely. When the lash is securely in place, apply a thin coat of eye liner directly to the lash line, toward the inner corner of the eye. Do not go all the way to the inside corner of the eye. This causes the liner to collect and form black dots in the corner, but more importantly, it makes the eye appear smaller.

Fake lashes must be cut to fit the eye. Although most are precut and feathered, the strip of lash is often too long for the eye and must be shortened from the outside end.

To remove the lash, grasp it firmly between your thumb and finger and remove it from the inside corner outward. Remove excess glue from your eye with eye makeup remover or by gently pulling it off with your fingers.

Another form of fake lashes is produced by tabbing—applying lashes in sets of one, two, or three, with glue, directly to the lash. This produces the most natural effect and, when applied properly, may last four to six weeks before all lashes need to be reaffixed.

Fake lashes must be kept clean and curled. Refer to Guide 3. Use alcohol to clean them. To curl them, wrap the lash around a pencil, wrap tissue or lightweight paper around the lash, and secure it with scotch tape or a rubber band. Allow several hours for the lash to recurl.

You will find fake lashes both fun and frustrating. One trick to help you enjoy fake lashes is to wear them daily for a week or more. Soon you will develop your own techniques for applying and removing your lashes. You may want to use tricks like those shown in Figures 36a through 36c. Again, practice with fake lashes before trying to wear them for the first time to an important nighttime

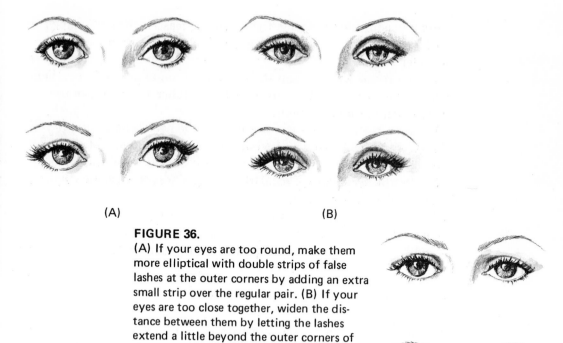

(A) **(B)**

FIGURE 36.
(A) If your eyes are too round, make them more elliptical with double strips of false lashes at the outer corners by adding an extra small strip over the regular pair. (B) If your eyes are too close together, widen the distance between them by letting the lashes extend a little beyond the outer corners of the eyes and by cutting off a few hairs at the inner corners. (C) If your eyes are too deep-set, make them more visible with a full, soft fringe of lashes, tapered to match your own but worn longer for emphasis.

(C)

affair or early morning interview. You may end up in a frenzied state with red watery eyes and ruin a good pair of eyelashes as well.

Another suggestion about your fake lashes: Experiment with an inexpensive pair from the dime store. This relieves the pressure of working with five-dollar lashes the first time around.

GUIDE 3

How To Make Lashes Last

1. When you remove lashes, hold them at one corner and gently ease them away from the lid. Put them back in their box to rest.
2. Remove adhesive build-up from the base by pulling it off gently with tweezers.
3. Clean the lashes, after several wearings, by rolling them over a

round pencil and brushing them with a mascara brush dampened with warm water. *Never* use cleaning fluid, and never immerse lashes in water.

4. To recurl lashes, wrap them around a round pencil, cover them with tissue paper, and secure it with a rubber band. *Never* use an eyelash curler on false lashes.

5. As a rule, mascara is not recommended for false lashes. If you do use it to blend lashes with your own, use a small amount.

6. Apply fixative carefully; don't let it spread onto eyelash hairs.

7. If you wear lashes regularly, equip yourself with two sets so that one pair can rest between wearings.

8. Always handle and store eyelashes carefully. Most are durable enough that you can flutter them all you wish, but tossing them around loosely in your handbag won't do much for their longevity.

LIP LOVELINESS

No picture would be complete without the perfect mouth and lip line. For some time now the lip has been ignored; in some cases not even a gloss has been worn by young American women. Color is returning to the scene. If you are blessed with vibrant, well-shaped lips, you can wear lip gloss for shine and proceed to other facets of beauty. However, over a period of time the lip loses this natural tone and must be indulged.

FIGURE 37.
(A) To shorten a wide mouth, stop lip outlines just short of the corners. (B) To widen a narrow mouth, extend the lip outline past the corners and use an upward tilt. (C) To make full lips narrower, outline inside the natural lipline with lipstick a shade lighter than your regular color. A too-full lower lip may be narrowed by using a darker shade of lipstick in the same color key. (D) Thin lips may be filled out by drawing outlines just outside the natural lipline, using a shade darker than your regular lipstick. (E) Lift the corners of a droopy mouth by tilting the outlines upward.

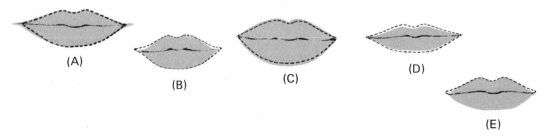

Shaping. Are your lips too thin, too thick, too long, too droopy, too narrow? See the illustrations of lip problems and methods to correct these problems in Figures 37a through 37e.

To reshape your lip line, you will first want to cover the entire lip, bottom and top, with foundation. Check that you have the correct tools for doing the job properly. The line must be perfectly smooth and formed, or the complete effect will be disastrous. Your tools are lipstick brush, red lip liner pencil, white lip liner pencil, lipstick, gloss, and powder.

Now begin with the red pencil liner; draw the desired shape of lip line, stopping your upper lip line short of the corner of the mouth. This prevents a drooping lip line effect.

If you have shortened the line or narrowed a full lower lip line, use the white pencil liner to work into the area of the lip outside the red line. This will cover the lip you do not want to color. When the perfect shape has been achieved—and this may take several tries—fill in the area within the red lip line.

Use the lipstick brush with your favorite shade of lipstick or a shade to complement your costume. Start at the points of the lip and work outward until the entire lip area is covered. Powder the lips and allow them to dry. Blot the lips and apply another coat of lipstick for a longer-lasting effect. Blot again and apply lip gloss. If you have never used a lip liner and lipstick brush, you will be thoroughly surprised with the effect and long-wearing results.

You have just completed the perfect picture. A great artist does not become great overnight; surely you will not expect to do so either. You must practice patiently and try many methods and products before you will become skillful enough to paint the perfect picture every time.

The products you use need not be the most expensive on the market. It is how you use them, not what you use! *Consumer Report*, a magazine available at most newsstands or by subscription, is an excellent source for finding listings of *pure* products available at the dime store.

The American woman is too well informed to be misled by advertising or packaging. She knows these costs are passed on to her in the price of the product. But there is a great psychological value to indulging in an expensive eye cream, moisturizer, or other new makeup product. It is a rewarding experience to experiment with makeup for today's look.

ENRICHMENT ACTIVITIES

1. Compile a notebook listing various skin care products you use regularly. Note products you find most effective for your particular skin type.

2. Make a study of the importance of diet and vitamins on skin. List the various groups of vitamins and note specific benefits of each for severe skin deficiencies and problems.

3. Set up a weekly skin care routine. Allow time for facials and other tension-easing skin routines, such as astringent-soaked cotton pads to soothe tired eyes or epsom salt soaks for weary feet.

4. Know which types of foods irritate your skin or make it appear too oily.

5. Prepare a book of beauty routines practiced by legendary women of great beauty and of beauty routines practiced by beautiful women today.

6. Study your particular skin type. Learn all you can about making it appear more lovely through the use of proper skin care routine, proper diet, exercise, and short rest periods during your busy day.

7. Make a habit of acquiring complimentary skin care pamphlets and gifts from cosmetic counters, drugstores, and doctors' offices.

8. Collect fashion shades of eye shadow, lipstick, and blushes of inexpensive brands. Experiment with these shades to enhance natural eye coloring and skin tone.

9. Collect brushes of all kinds—art brushes, tooth brushes, complexion brushes, shadow brushes, and others—to use in applying your makeup. Brushes are easy to work with and prevent stretching of facial tissue.

10. Analyze your brow line to be sure it complements your facial structure. Do not draw on the line. Shorten the brow line if your forehead is narrow; lengthen the brow line if your forehead is broad. Be sure your brow color blends with your hair color; never should your brow be *much* darker or *much* lighter than your hair.

success secrets for
beautiful hands and feet

The role your hands and feet play in projecting your visible image should never be underestimated. After all, you "speak with your hands," wave hello to friends, and type that VIP letter, while your feet propel you along to new adventures. Hands, especially nails, are continually on display, and feet, whether bare or in strappy sandals, are almost as much so. Without a doubt, a beautiful manicure and pedicure are a plus for greater self-confidence and good looks.

Today's woman would hardly argue that nail and hand care are not important, but the two points she is most concerned about are: "What are the basic essentials of hand care?" and "How can I give myself a quick, professional looking manicure that will last?"

Habitual, continuing hand care is important. If a well-done manicure calls attention to rough, grimy, reddened, or poorly kept hands, then the effect of the manicure is wasted.

HAND CARE HABITS

These practical suggestions, faithfully observed, will reward you with hands that always look their best.

1. Hand cream or lotion should be used before and after wet or messy jobs. Wear rubber gloves whenever possible.

2. Try an occasional all-night beauty treatment by massaging face cream or rich oil (olive or baby oil) over your hands. Massage by working the skin of the fingers and hand toward the wrist as though putting on gloves. Work each finger separately, starting with the right hand. Repeat with the left hand. Use this same motion when applying lotion. Wear roomy cotton gloves to protect your sheets.

3. To remove cooking odors, splash on vinegar and rinse in cold water.

4. Bleach stains or discolorations with a cut lemon, the cut side of a raw potato, or with oatmeal rubbed on wet hands.

5. Before gardening, polishing furniture, painting, or doing other dirty tasks, dig your nails into a bar of wet soap. Later the soil will wash away easily.

6. If your hands perspire, try patting them with skin freshener or a cologne, or spray them with antiperspirant.

7. To give emergency first aid to rough, red hands, mix a tablespoon of granulated sugar with a bit of olive or baby oil and work the mixture gently into the hands. Soaking hands for ten minutes in a mixture of lemon juice and baby oil is also effective.

EXERCISES FOR EXPRESSIVE HANDS

Hands are just like the rest of the body—the more you exercise them, the more graceful they become. Natural, relaxed gestures soon become second nature.

The simple exercises, shown in Figures 38 through 41, contribute to expressive hand movements. In addition, they help to eliminate tension in arm and shoulder muscles.

NAIL KNOWLEDGE

There is no dodging the issue! Pretty nails on well-groomed hands are an important part of your total beauty picture. As a background for proper nail care, study and understand the formation of your nails as detailed in Figure 42. The visible nail is a hard plate that begins in the nail matrix. The matrix is located at the base of the nail with

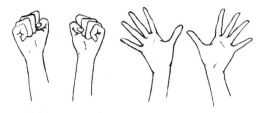

FIGURE 38.
Place your elbows on a table, make your hands into fists, then open your hands and spread the fingers apart.

FIGURE 39.
Pretend you are typing a letter or playing the piano. Lift each finger separately.

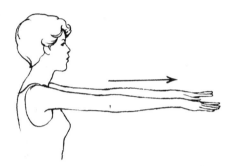

FIGURE 40.
Hold your hands and arms stiffly out in front of you. Relax and loosen them. Shake them so your fingers fly.

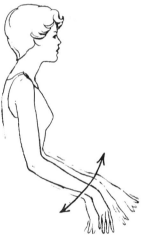

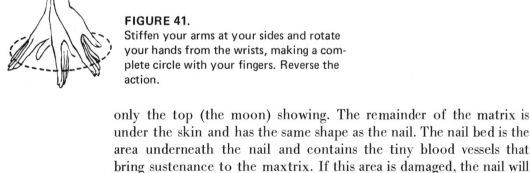

FIGURE 41.
Stiffen your arms at your sides and rotate your hands from the wrists, making a complete circle with your fingers. Reverse the action.

only the top (the moon) showing. The remainder of the matrix is under the skin and has the same shape as the nail. The nail bed is the area underneath the nail and contains the tiny blood vessels that bring sustenance to the maxtrix. If this area is damaged, the nail will have a defect until it grows out. Good nails and a good matrix go hand in hand, and this is why you must be careful not to bruise or cut the base of the nail.

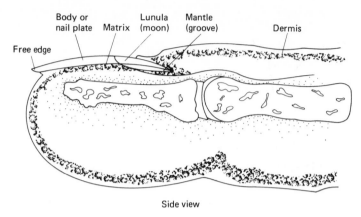

Body or
nail plate   Lunula   Mantle
nail plate Matrix (moon) (groove)   Dermis

Free edge

Side view

FIGURE 42.
Nail section.

The question, "Can I increase the rate of nail growth?" is often asked. Perhaps. The nails on the hand you use most and the middle nails of both hands grow faster than those fingers that receive less use. They also grow faster during pregnancy and youth. Activities such as typing and piano playing promote more rapid growth, as do buffing and massaging the fingertips to improve circulation. Anything that causes you to use your hands more will influence more rapid growth.

Although seldom recognized, emotions are a factor in general nail health. Like skin and hair, nails reflect your state of health. For example, during surgery the nails are indicators of blood circulation. Because of this, a lot of beautiful presurgery manicures and pedicures have to be removed. To test circulation, the doctor presses lightly on the nail, then watches to see how quickly the blood returns. You may apply this same test to get a general idea of how adequate the blood circulation to your nails is.

Have you ever wondered what the various marks on your nails mean? Faint lines running from cuticle to nail tip indicate dryness and usually occur in older people. Horizontal ridges, alike on all nails, generally indicate an illness in the not too distant past. Small white spots, scattered at random on the nails, show that the person is suffering from frazzled nerves and tension. They may also result from severe emotional upset or a disease.

The effect of proper diet on the appearance of hands and nails cannot be emphasized strongly enough. For example, nutritional deficiencies can cause nails to be too soft. Lack of iodine is a common cause of weak nails that split and break. Your dietary iodine supply can be increased by eating seafood or by taking seaweed (kelp) in capsule form. Several months after the addition of a daily kelp tablet to the diet, most people are amazed at the improvement in the strength and appearance of their nails. A colorless form of iodine can be painted directly onto the nails and is also very beneficial. Some cuticle creams contain white iodine; ask for this type when you buy.

Another cause of splits and breaks is protein deficiency. This may be solved by the addition of a daily gelatin drink to your diet. Tests have shown that a daily envelope of unflavored gelatin mixed with juice or a hot drink (or flavored gelatin mixed with water) will clear up or drastically improve problem nails within three to five months. Patience is necessary as the minimum "grow-out" period of nails is three months. After adding the gelatin to your diet you may also notice a marked improvement in the texture and quality of your hair and skin as they too are directly affected by the protein in your diet.

Less known, but just as important, is the value of calcium. Nails actually use more of this mineral than the skin or hair. Frequently, additional vitamin A will also improve the quality of the nails.

FEET FACTS

It has been said, "When your feet hurt, you hurt all over," and "An ounce of prevention is worth a pound of cure." Painful foot problems can be prevented by following these suggestions.

1. Improperly fitting, uncomfortable, or tight shoes can make you irritable and bad-tempered. The unmistakable clue to a flaw in fit is a rubbed, red spot anywhere on your feet.
2. When you buy shoes, have both feet measured while you are standing. Put on both shoes, stand up, and walk around. The tip of your longest toe should be one-half to three-quarters of an inch from the end of the shoe.
3. Too tight or too short hose can cause foot problems in the same way improperly fitting shoes do.
4. Corns, callouses, or hard places should *never* be cut or shaved. Smooth them with a pumice stone, emery board, or an abrasive grooming powder.

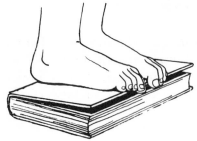

FIGURE 43.
Place your bare foot on a book and repeatedly curl
your toes over the edge. This relaxing exercise is
designed for tired, aching feet. It also strengthens
the arch.

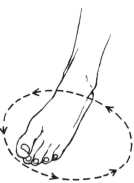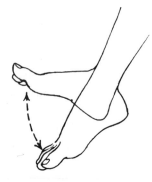

FIGURE 44.
Hold the leg out straight and move the foot in a circular motion. Then move it
up and down. This exercise is designed to strengthen and relax the ankle.

5. Spray deodorant powders are excellent for clammy,
   perspiring feet. Talcum powder sprinkled in just-worn
   shoes will absorb the moisture.

6. Athlete's foot (watery blisters and thick white skin
   between toes) should be treated by a doctor. If you have
   this highly contagious disease, do not walk barefoot where
   you might expose other people.

7. Corns, ingrown toenails, callouses, or other abnormal
   conditions should be treated by a podiatrist or chiropodist.

8. Even when shoes fit properly, nasty little pressure areas
   may develop. To prevent a corn or callous from forming,
   cover the area with moleskin or lamb's wool.

9. Treat feet to frequent massages. Rub in hand cream, baby
   oil, or rich night cream, using a rotating, kneading motion.
   Work it in from the heel up to the knee and then tug and
   work it into the toes. Occasionally apply a heavy coat of
   lubricant and sleep in cotton socks. These few minutes of
   extra care will pay handsome dividends in terms of snagless
   hose and soft, feminine feet.

10. First aid for fatigued feet may be acquired by lying on the bed or floor and putting the feet up against a wall for a few minutes. A bicarbonate of soda footbath does double duty as a skin softener and fatigue reliever. Dissolve two tablespoons of bicarbonate of soda in a basin of warm water, and soak your feet.

11. Go barefoot whenever possible. The air and sunshine are very healthy.

EXERCISES FOR FEMININE FEET

The exercises shown in Figures 43 and 44 may be performed under cover of your desk as a work or study break.

THE NAIL CARE KIT

Organization, the key to fast, efficient accomplishment of any task, applies particularly to the manicure-pedicure routine. The idea is to work out a streamlined system that will keep hands and feet looking their best in a minimum amount of time.

It is important to assemble a kit that contains all the equipment and materials needed. You might wish to cover a small box with bright adhesive paper or decorate a cute basket to hold the essentials. Needless to say, when manicure time comes, minutes will not be wasted while you search for supplies. The kit should include:

Emery board, seven or eight inches long, or a diamond-dust file
Orangewood cuticle stick
Nail brush
Cuticle nippers (optional)
Cuticle scissors
Nail buffer (optional)
Oily polish remover
Absorbent cotton
Cotton swabs
Cuticle remover
Cuticle cream (should contain white iodine)
White vinegar
Base coat (one containing protein helps strengthen nails)

Nail polish
Colorless topcoat
A fast-dry spray (optional)

MANICURE PROCEDURE

Hands are said to "speak," and they actually do. Beautifully kept nails serve as the exclamation points of the hands! To keep those exclamation points sharply in focus, a good manicure every week or ten days is necessary. If you do your nails correctly, you won't be forced to waste precious minutes in repair work throughout the week. Learn the right procedure and then perform it smoothly and speedily. For a perfect manicure:

1. Remove old polish. Use a cotton square moistened (not soaked) in remover. Press it against the nail for a few seconds, then bring the pad down firmly from the base of the nail. Do not smear the old polish into the cuticle or onto the fingers.

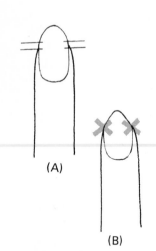

(A)

(B)

FIGURE 45.

2. Shape the nails to graceful ovals of approximately the same medium length. File them with an emery board or a diamond-dust file. Never use a plain metal file because the metal encourages splitting. To develop nail strength, let the sides grow out square a sixteenth to an eighth of an inch from the nail base, as illustrated in Figure 45a. Never file deep into the nail corners as shown in Figure 45b. To file properly, hold your hand flat on a table with your fingers pointing away from you. File gently with the coarse side of a file or emery board slanting from underneath the nail. Use short, one-way strokes from sides to center, being careful not be bevel the nail edges. Nails are formed in layers, and a beveled edge leaves some layers protruding. The smallest pressure will cause these layers to separate and start a troublesome peeling cycle. Filing should always be done from underneath the nail, never from the top.

3. Apply cuticle remover with a cotton swab. Work it thoroughly around the edges of the nails.

4. Using a cotton-wrapped orange stick, push the cuticle back gently until the base of the nail is as square as possible. A squared base, as shown in Figure 46, provides a strong

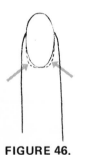

FIGURE 46.

foundation for nail growth; if you do not bite or pick at your fingers, hangnails will soon be eliminated.

5. With the flat end of the orange stick, lift the cuticle rim very gently and clean away traces of dead tissue. Work lightly, from the base to the tip of the nail, being careful not to bruise the nail base.

6. Clean under the free edge. Use a cotton swab dipped in soapy water, cuticle oil, or hydrogen peroxide.

7. Soak the nails in warm, soapy water; then use a nail brush to scrub away loose cuticle.

8. Trim hangnails only if absolutely necessary. Try to avoid cutting cuticles; they become tougher and generally more ragged. If a cut should occur while you are trimming the cuticle, swab it with hydrogen peroxide or alcohol.

9. Apply cuticle cream. Gently massage it in, using a rotating movement with the thumb of the opposite hand.

10. To remove the cream, again immerse the nails in warm, soapy water and brush them with a downward movement.

11. Clean away remaining traces of oil and soap with a cotton square moistened in white vinegar. Let the nails dry. This step is important because it insures that your polish will adhere tightly.

12. Brush on a base coat, preferably one that contains protein.

13. Apply polish in three smooth, quick strokes, beginning at the cuticle and sweeping to the nail tip. Do the center first, then the sides. Let the first coat dry (it takes about five minutes); then apply the second coat. There should be just enough polish on your brush to do one nail without redipping. If the polish thickens, thin it with solvent and shake it well. Avoid touching the cuticle with polish. Remove it with a cotton-tipped orange stick if the polish does get onto the cuticle.

14. Brush a colorless, sealing top coat over the nail and under the tip.

15. Use fast-dry spray if you wish.

FINGER TIPS

These principles of nail care and maintenance make a vital contribution to the overall appearance of your hands.

1. To protect your manicure:
    a. Use a pencil when dialing the telephone.
    b. Learn to use the cushion of your fingers when picking things up.
    c. To work light switches, elevator buttons, and door bells, use the knuckle of your index finger.
2. If nail biting is a problem, give yourself a really super manicure and then resolve each day not to bite your nails until the next day. It's easier to make it one day at a time.
3. If nails are splitting and peeling, buff them gently to strengthen and bind the edges.
4. Do not peel off polish because this weakens nails.
5. To repair a broken or split nail, brush on a base coat or colorless sealer, then place a tiny piece of nail mending tissue (facial tissue may be substituted) over the break as shown in Figure 47. Tuck the tissue under the edge, smooth it, and apply one or two more coats of the base or sealer. Nail mending kits can be purchased.

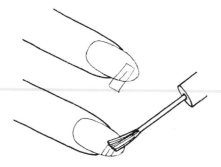

FIGURE 47.
Repair of a broken or split nail.

FIGURE 48.
Correct polishing for the four basic nail types.

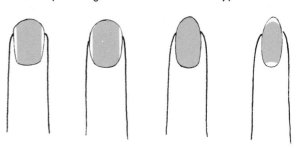

6. Use care in deciding to use false nails. You may be allergic to the glue or may damage your own nails. If you do decide to use them, check the glue on one nail first.

7. Never file nails after they have been in water. Wet nails are weak and subject to splitting.

8. Don't blow on your nails or hold them in front of an air conditioning or heating vent to speed drying. The polish will dry too fast on the surface, and bubbles will form underneath. Bubbles may also appear if you use too thick a coat of polish.

9. Repair chipped polish as soon as possible.

10. Nails that are too long can look like claws. Try to keep your nails approximately the same length.

11. Polish color can create a corrective illusion. Light polish makes nails appear delicate. Dark shades make nails appear smaller. Medium shades make nails look larger.

12. To improve the appearance of broad, spatulate, or narrow nails, polish is applied as shown in Figure 48.

FOR A PERFECT PEDICURE

In polishing your toenails, the method is similar to that of a manicure. To avoid ingrown toenails, cut and file nails straight across. Should ingrown nails occur, clip a "V" in the center of the toenail tip to relieve the pressure. Keep nails shorter than the ends of your toes and do not cut the corners. Brush polish over the edge of the nail, not only because it's prettier but because it makes a smoother finish that is less likely to snag hose. To keep polish from smudging, separate the toes with little rolls of cotton or tissue. Keep your feet smooth by using pumice stone or abrasive powder and by massaging them often with hand lotion or cream.

Remember: The reward of extra self-confidence you reap when you know your hands, nails, and feet are well cared for will be worth the effort you put in to learning and practicing the secrets of successful manicure/pedicure routines.

ENRICHMENT ACTIVITIES

1. Decorate a container to hold your manicure/pedicure essentials.

2. Accumulate the necessary items to fully stock your manicure kit.

3. Resolve to give yourself a manicure and pedicure once every week or ten days.

4. When next you have a broken or split nail, practice mending it with tissue.

5. Observe the manner in which your friends file their nails. If they are filing incorrectly, you can share with them what you have learned.

6. Share with friends nail tips that you have learned in this chapter.

7. Begin drinking one package of gelatin daily.

8. Start a file of newspaper and magazine clippings that relate to hand and foot care.

9. Check any of the following bad habits with which you are troubled. Resolve to correct them.

Nail biting
Continual hand waving while you are talking
Picking cuticles
Peeling nail polish
Never drinking milk
Removing polish several times a week
Allowing nails to be different lengths, running the course from very short to very long, all on the same hand

poise
in motion

Poise is elusive and mysterious. It is a mental attitude that gives a woman self-confidence so that she can meet all situations with grace, compassion, and dignity.

Visual poise could also be called body language—the way a woman creates moods, communicates, and draws people to her. She can set the mood for a person or group of people by the flow of her walk, the softness of her voice, and the tenderness of her gesture.

The effectiveness of woman's charm and poise is recorded throughout history. Samson cut his hair for Delilah, Romeo gave his last devoted breath for Juliet, and the Duke of Windsor abdicated his throne for the love of his life.

You can make history too! With concentrated effort you can acquire self-confidence, composure, bearing, and dignity.

Right now, while reading this book—freeze—don't move. Take a good look at yourself. What about *your* posture? Are you slumped over a desk with your feet wrapped around the chair legs; do you have a crick in your neck? Maybe you've been there for quite a while and you need to exercise; so please get up and walk to a full-length mirror, and take a good look at yourself. Stand the way you usually stand and look at yourself from the front and from the side. You may see some figure faults that can be corrected with good posture. You can convey to people much about your self-esteem by the way you move and carry your body. If you stand tall, hold your head high, and glide when you walk, you are saying to people you meet that you have confidence in yourself and can handle the situation. On the other hand, if you slump, have awkward, jerky movements and a clumsy walk, you give the impression of being moody and having an inferiority complex.

In a self-improvement program, posture is the foundation on which to build visual poise. Practicing correct posture can make you an inch taller, or help you to have confidence in your height if you are tall. It will give you a smaller waist, a flatter tummy, and diminish your derriére. Your clothes will fit better because they are designed for figures with everything in the right places. You will have better control of your muscles and less "jello." Correct posture will even eliminate back pains caused from strained muscles, aid your digestive tract, and make you more alert because you will take the wrinkles out of your lungs. It will bring you untold dividends because you will take your eyes from the dust and dirt of the sidewalk and look up and smile at people passing by. And your smile will cause someone else to smile, and that is called "Smile Pollution." We would like to see more of that, wouldn't you? And just think—all of this is yours if you have concern for yourself. It won't cost you a penny; but it will cost you some time and effort.

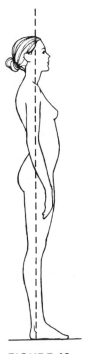

FIGURE 49.

BE OBJECTIVE

It is difficult to be objective in performing a self-analysis. To improve your posture, you should try to see yourself as you are. Some women don't take constructive criticism too well, especially from a friend. And who would want to ask a friend to list all of one's weak points? The task is yours. Figure 49 shows a woman with posture problems; how many are yours?

It is good to write thoughts down; it seems to make a stronger impression. To execute a self-analysis effectively, you must try to appraise yourself as you would a stranger. To start, fill in the Visual Poise Analysis shown in Chart 1.

Believe it or not, a camera is your friend. I don't mean one in a studio with filters and soft lights, but rather the kind you or your friends use. Have two ordinary full-length pictures taken, one of you squarely facing the camera and one of your profile. Wear a dress, knee-length or shorter, that has a waist or an illusion of a waist. Have three-by-five-inch pictures made of each pose, and paste them into

CHART 1

Visual Poise Analysis

Posture _____

_____

_____

Good or needs attention? List strong and weak points.

Body Muscle Tone _____

_____

_____

Firm or relaxed? If you are a combination, determine how to firm your relaxed muscles, face and neck included.

Body Language _____

_____

_____

Do you reflect self-esteem and poise, or insecurity and awkwardness?

Mannerisms _____

_____

_____

Do you constantly run your fingers through your hair, bite your lip, blink your eyelashes excessively, or continually adjust your clothes or look in a mirror?

Posture Problems or Bad Habits

Do you have any of the following?

Swayback	Toeing in or out when you walk
Dowager hump	Shuffling or bouncing walk
Drooping shoulders	Swinging arms when you walk
Caved in chest	Moving upper torso when you walk
Sagging stomach	Bending at the waist when you
Leading chin when you walk	stoop
Arms folded across your rib section	Knees apart when you sit
	Stiff knees when you stand
Slumping and slouching	A habit of collapsing into a chair

your workbook. This is a good beginning; you can see your assets and liabilities.

Place a piece of tracing paper over the pictures, Figures 50 and 51, and trace your silhouettes. For the silhouette facing the camera, with a ruler, draw a line vertically through the center of the body. Now draw a perpendicular line exactly at shoulders, waist, and hips. Is your body equally distributed on either side of the vertical line? Are your shoulders, hips, and waist on both sides of your body touching the horizontal lines? If not, you are higher on one side than the other. Is your bust line half the distance between your shoulder and elbow?

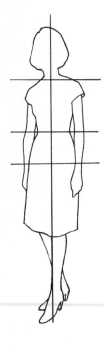

FIGURE 50.
Trace the silhouette of your picture facing the camera, and analyze it.

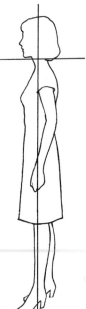

FIGURE 51.
Trace the silhouette of your profile, and analyze it.

Do the same exercise with your profile, and check the same points with the following additions. Is your chin parallel with the floor, and are you swaybacked? Refer to Figures 50 and 51 when you perform this exercise.

At this time it will be wise to take all of your measurements. The measurements should include your vital statistics (bust, waist, hips) as well as your diaphragm, the distance between your last rib and the top of your hip bone, thighs, calves, and the length of your waist. Record this information on a chart for a permanent record. You will need to refer to this later in the course.

Another exercise to perform, possibly in the classroom, is with

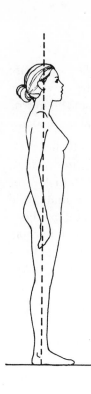

FIGURE 52.
The spine is a rod or plumb line through the middle of the body. Think tall, stand tall, feel tall, walk tall, and sit tall.

a plumb line. Attach a cord, with a metal bob tied to the end, to the ceiling or the top of a door opening. Stand perpendicular to the cord. If your body alignment is correct, the cord will bisect your body through your ear lobe, neck, shoulder joint, elbow, waist, wrist, hip, back of knee, and ankle as shown in Figure 52.

You now have a visual picture of your posture profile and can see what needs special attention. Your spine is a rod or plumb line, and if it is straight, you have passed the test.

After you have worked on correcting your posture for several months, have another set of pictures made, and perform all of the above experiments again. You will be delighted at the difference in your posture and figure.

SEVEN STEPS TO GOOD POSTURE

Practicing good posture all the time is like exercising all the time. It is very important that each part of your body—feet, legs, torso, spine, and head—stack up in their proper places as shown in Figure 53. Here are the seven steps to good posture.

Feet Flat on the Floor. Your feet are your foundation and the balance for your body. The weight of your body should be over the arch and ball of your foot. When you are standing, you should be able to lift your heels off the floor and wiggle your toes simultaneously. If your body weight is on your heels, you will settle too far back and this will cause you to lose your balance easily.

Relaxed Knees. When someone says, "Stand up straight," it doesn't mean to click your heels together and lock your knees. Locked, tight knees can be the cause of bad posture because they throw the rest of the body completely out of line. Rather, the knees should be relaxed with a natural bend. Just as your elbows have a natural bend when relaxed at your side, so do the knees when you are standing properly.

Try this exercise. Stand sideways in front of a full-length mirror; lock your knees and see what happens to your posture. Your legs will have a bow and your derrière will be out way too far. In this

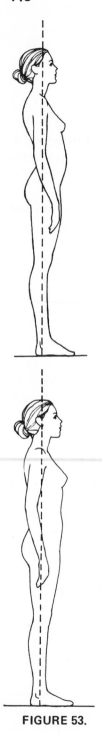

FIGURE 53.

position, your posture is extremely swaybacked. If locked knees are a natural position for you, start correcting the bad habit now. This can be done by simply relaxing the knees. As you look in the mirror and relax your knees, notice what happens to your legs and buttocks.

Hips Tucked Under. The American woman seems to be more concerned with her hips than almost any part of her figure; in fact, she is extremely sensitive about them. If you will learn to tuck your hips under, you can diminish your derrière. Tuck them under and pinch the muscles very hard at the same time. This is a good exercise: Imagine you are trying to get out of your car on a crowded parking lot, and your car door will open just a few inches. In order to get out you will try to make yourself as small as possible by tucking under and then tightening all of your muscles.

Stomach Pulled In. Perhaps one of the most common figure destroyers is a protruding abdomen, the stomach spilling out of the pelvis. When you did the previous exercise, it did wonders for your stomach, too. If the hips are tucked under, the pelvic area is tilted back, where it belongs, and this helps to make the stomach smaller. The following exercise is rewarding: Stand as you normally do; with a tape measure take your stomach measurement four inches down from your waistline. Now tuck under and tighten your hip and stomach muscles, and measure yourself again. How much difference is there in the two measurements? As you continue to practice this and make it a natural part of your daily posture, the muscles will become tight and firm.

Rib Cage Pulled Up and Out of Waist. Who doesn't want an inch-smaller waist! Many women are guilty of letting their ribs rest on their hip bones, and this causes a "spare tire" around the middle. Stretching is good for the body and should be a natural part of posture. Pull your rib cage up and out of your hips, and stretch the waist area. It not only helps to make the waist smaller, it also will increase your height; you may be an inch taller. As you stretch taller you will be amazed at the deep breaths you take, possibly the first in a long time. The wrinkles will come out of your lungs and they will completely fill with oxygen. Deep breathing is good to relieve nervous tension and will help you keep mentally alert.

Shoulders Back and Relaxed. Pull your shoulders up and back, with your blades almost touching, and now down and relaxed. This will lift your breasts high, where they belong; put your neck in the proper position, with your ear lobes centered over your shoulders; and your arms will fall at your sides with the palms turned in against your body. You should not look stiff, but relaxed. Practice will make this possible.

Chin Up and Parallel with the Floor. When you hold your head high, don't lift your nose and throw your chin up high, which makes you look snooty. Rather, imagine you have a string attached to each ear, like a puppet, and lift your head by pulling up on the strings. This will give a stretching, uplifting feeling, and your chin will be parallel with the floor.

Most women have two chins, but it certainly isn't fashionable or flattering to show them. Notice how many people in the public eye have acquired the habit of holding the head high with dignity.

To get the feel of the Seven Steps to Good Posture that you have just read, stand next to a wall with your feet about two inches away from the wall and perform the exercise in Figure 54. Press your head, shoulders, back, and hips hard against the wall. If you can slide your hand between the wall and the small of your back, you are too swaybacked. In order to press all of your vertebrae against the wall, bend your knees and slide down the wall until your entire back touches it. Press hard, return to the standing position, and walk away from the wall. Now your body is in perfect alignment. At first this

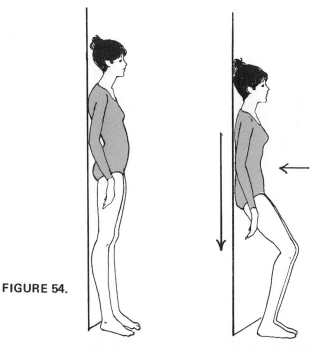

FIGURE 54.

may seem strange, but with practice it will feel natural and become a part of you.

The following exercise (in Figure 55) is also good for strengthening your posture.

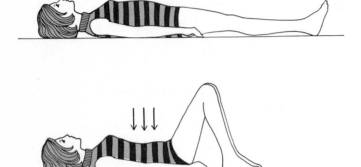

FIGURE 55.

1. Lie on your back on the floor.
2. Bend your knees until your feet are flat on the floor.
3. Press with your stomach muscles until your back touches the floor, hold, and release. Repeat five to ten times daily.

Take advantage of any spare time you have to exercise. When you are riding in a car or sitting in a chair, let the time work for your good posture. Press your back against the seat back until all of your spine is touching the seat, hold, and release. This exercise will strengthen stomach and back muscles needed for correct posture.

STAND TALL

Standing correctly is the sum total of the Seven Steps to Good Posture, and the exercises that accompany them. Practice these steps to put yourself together in the correct standing position. It is very important to work in front of a mirror. As you face the mirror straight on, you will see that your body has a blocky look. For your stance to be graceful, you must angle your body slightly, so it will fall into a triangular shape.

Take a lesson from models, and learn the hesitation stance. Stand with one foot slightly behind the other. The back foot should be about two inches behind the front foot and turned at a slight angle. Relax the knee of the front leg, with the toes straight ahead. The back foot should bear most of the weight. The front knee will overlap the back knee. Twist your hips slightly in the direction of the back foot. You will look five pounds slimmer. Now turn from your waist and look straight ahead. Let your arms fall naturally at your side with a little separation at your waist. The hand on the side of your body that has the foot back should fall slightly in front of your side seam, and vice versa. This pose will show your legs at their prettiest no matter what their shape. Figure 56 shows that the look is one of composure and lightness, not the military look with both feet apart and plunked straight ahead.

You may feel awkward when you first try the hesitation stance, but practice it until it becomes a beautiful habit.

When you are standing, you don't always have to leave your hands at your sides. Here are three other hand positions you may try:

1. With your elbows slightly bent to allow space between your arms and body, clasp your fingers in front, holding them just below your waist.
2. You can assume the same position with your hands in back.
3. Cross your arms and rest one hand above the elbow, and the other hand on the elbow of the other arm.

WALK GRACEFULLY

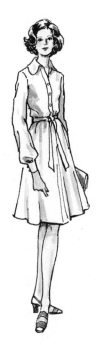

A woman with a smooth, graceful walk commands attention and admiration. By contrast, a woman with jerky movements, slumped over, and leading with her chin is not enviable. The career model attracts attention with her smooth, almost floating glide as few other women are able to do. However, remember that she has been practicing and making it a natural part of her poise for a long, long time. It will take you many hours of determined practice to master the art of walking gracefully.

FIGURE 56.
The hesitation stance: Body and feet are in three-quarter position.

A graceful walk depends on good posture. Everything you have studied to this point has prepared you for walking. You will want to move with as little unnecessary motion as possible. Your body must be aligned with head held high, shoulders back and relaxed, arms at your sides, stomach in, buttocks tucked under, knees relaxed, and toes straight ahead.

Maintaining your perfect body posture, step forward with your left foot. The movement should come from your hip joints, not the knees. Keep your knees slightly flexed to act as shock absorbers when your feet touch the floor.

Your heel does not touch the floor first. This causes a hard, jerky movement. With your toes pointed straight ahead, the ball of your foot touches the floor first; and your heel touches immediately. In very slow motion it would be toe, ball, heel. As the ball of your foot touches the floor, your weight change begins by lifting the heel of the back foot and giving a little push with the toes. Figure 57 shows the movements in slow motion.

As you walk, your knees may graze one another. Your steps should create two parallel lines about two inches apart. It would be very good to practice walking along two pieces of tape placed on the floor, or on a hardwood floor where you see the lines of the wood. Practice to music that has a slow, rhythmic beat. Keep a stride that is

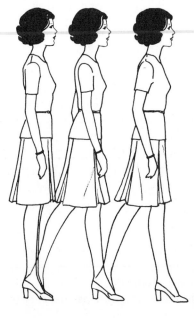

FIGURE 57.
A graceful walk depends on good posture. Move with as little unnecessary motion as possible.

in proportion with your body. It should be about the length of your foot. If the stride is too long, you will have a bouncy, masculine walk, and if it is too short you will have the stiff walk of an old lady.

There should be some motion in your hands as you walk, but they should not fly in the air. Your fingertips will lightly brush the fabric of the garment you are wearing. Your right hand and left foot will come forward at the same time. Practice your walk to eliminate excess motion. The upper torso, from your hip to the top of your head, should have no motion. Keep the hip movement at a minimum. Place your hands on your hips; if your elbows move, you have too much movement in your hips.

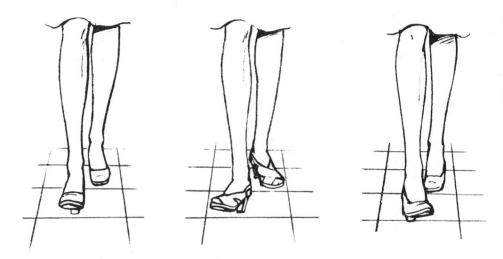

FIGURE 58.
Point your toes straight ahead when you walk. Don't toe in or out.

Do you realize that your walk has a personality? How many times have you been busy and without looking up said, "Here comes Sue." How did you know it was Sue? You recognized her walk. Some walks have a shuffle, a dragging shoe, a hard touch. Every graceful walk has rhythm. The sound of feet on the floor should be quiet and smooth.

Your shoes will tell you a lot about your walk. Look at the soles and the bottom of the heels. If you are not holding your feet straight, the shoes will be run over and one side of the sole will be more worn than the other. Hitting the floor heavily with your heels first will cause the back of the heel caps to wear down rapidly. Do you have black scuff marks on the insides of your shoes? This means you are slinging your heels in and toes out as you walk. You can eliminate these marks by pointing your toes straight. Refer to Figure 58 for correct and incorrect toe positions.

SIT PRETTY

More personal appearances have been destroyed by the lack of grace when a woman sits than you may realize. Some women flop into the big comfortable-looking easy chairs only to find that there is no way out without performing acrobatics. And there are those who never keep their knees together and cause lots of embarrassment for everyone concerned. How many times have you had to sit and look at someone's stocking tops and girdle? Figure 59 shows how these incidents can destroy a feminine image.

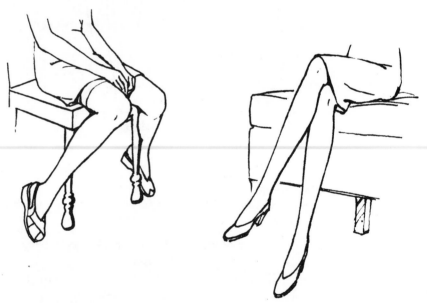

FIGURE 59.
Keep your knees and ankles together when you sit.

Sitting pretty is simple once you have mastered the art of approaching, sitting on, and leaving a chair. When you enter a room and there is a choice of chairs, lounge or straight, select the straight chair. They are easier to handle with poise and grace. Before you can master the approach to a chair, you need to learn the turn, or pivot. There are three steps involved.

1. Step forward with your right foot and keep the ball of your left foot on the floor, with the heel slightly raised.
2. Lift your right heel off the floor. Now your weight is balanced on the balls of both feet.
3. With your weight forward, turn to the left and face the opposite direction. Assume the natural standing position: both feet on the floor with the balance of body weight on the back foot, which is angled, and the lead foot slightly forward with the toes straight ahead.

Approach the chair straight on, and just before you get there, turn. When you turn, the calf of your lead foot will touch the chair, and you will know the chair is there. You will not have to turn around and reassure yourself of its presence. Lower your body onto the edge of the chair using your thigh and calf muscles. Keep your

FIGURE 60.
Master the art of sitting gracefully.

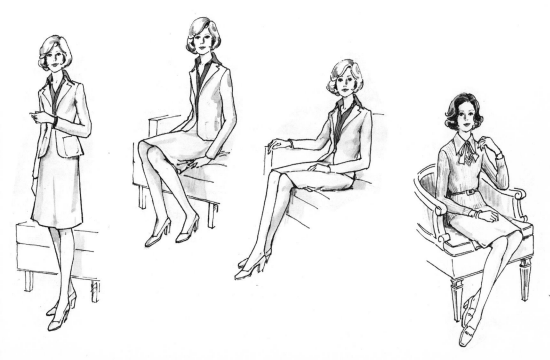

head up, back straight, and your buttocks tucked under. With your hands close to your body and placed on the edge of the chair, lift your body up slightly and move to the back of the chair. Sit at an angle in the chair; this will give your body an "S" curve. Figure 60 shows correct body positions.

To leave the chair, reverse your movements. Keeping your torso straight, place one foot slightly under the chair, and use your leg muscles to lift your body gracefully. Don't rely on the chair arms to help you in or out of a chair.

Don't be guilty of always crossing your legs; there are several other leg positions for you to learn. Please remember that whatever you do with your feet, always keep your knees together. This is of cardinal importance to sitting prettily. If you keep your back straight, your knees will touch; if you slump, your knees will separate—try it. Try other positions:

1. Place your feet flat on the floor, and bring the heel of one foot to rest at the instep of the other foot.
2. Sitting at an angle in a chair, place one foot behind the other, crossing them at the ankles, and keep your toes pointed in the same direction. Now pull your feet back under the edge of the chair. If your body is angled to the right of the chair, arrange your feet at the left with the right foot behind the left one.
3. Cross your legs at the ankles or the knees. When crossing your legs cross them high above the knees, with your lower legs parallel. Angle your legs to the side, and keep the toes of both feet pointed toward the floor.

The following are several hand positions you can rely on for confidence and poise while you are sitting:

1. Place one hand on your lap, palm down, and gently lay the other hand on top of it or on the wrist.
2. Lay one hand in your lap, palm up, and lay the other hand in it, palm up, and clasp your fingers gently.
3. Place both hands on their sides, little fingers against your leg; gently entwine your fingers with your thumbs crossed on top.

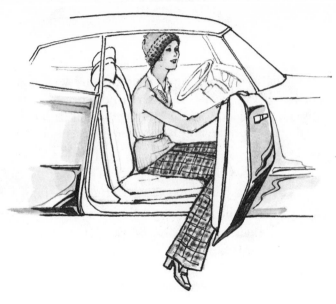

FIGURE 61.
Don't crawl into a car. Sit on the seat first, and then move in.

THE CHALLENGE OF THE AUTOMOBILE

Entering and leaving cars is one of the most difficult movements to perform gracefully because cars come in all sizes and shapes. Please remember that one never crawls into a car. Practice the following procedures shown in Figure 61 and you will meet the challenge.

1. Stand as close to the car as possible with the side of your body next to the seat.
2. Sit down on the edge of the seat first. Head and feet are still out of the car.
3. Swing your feet into the car, keeping your knees together, moving your body and head in at the same time.
4. After your body is in the car, move over on the seat and arrange your skirt.

When you leave the car:

1. Your body and feet go out first, keeping your knees together.
2. When your feet touch the ground, bend over from the waist. As you move your body out of the car, return to the standing position as smoothly as possible.

This is the method of entering and leaving a car that has been practiced for years. However, because of changes in fashions, lifestyle, and automobile designs, the following procedure has become acceptable and is practiced by many knowledgeable women.

1. Stand beside the open door, facing forward.
2. Rest your outer hand on the inside door handle.
3. Put the foot nearest the car in first.
4. Bend your knees, keeping them together, and slide your buttocks in.
5. Carefully lift your other leg and the rest of your body into the car, and move back on the seat.

The techniques of visual poise require the use of the leg muscles, balance, time, and perseverance. You will feel awkward at first, but keep practicing until you feel natural, gain self-confidence, and attract admiring glances.

ENRICHMENT ACTIVITIES

1. Perform all of the exercises listed in the chapter.
2. Record your measurements: height, weight, bust, waist, hip, thighs, calves.
3. Practice the Seven Steps to Good Posture daily.
4. Stand correctly, and try different graceful hand positions.
5. Practice walking in front of a mirror every day.
6. Have someone help you analyze your walk.
7. Practice the hesitation stance.
8. Perform the posture exercises daily.
9. Listen for different walking personalities.
10. Check your shoes for tips about your walk.
11. List all of your posture problems in standing, walking, and sitting, and determine how you will correct each one.

in trim with the times

One of the most widely discussed topics in the United States and throughout the world today is *diet*. There are many myths related to diet—various "crash" or "unusual" routines that result in overnight success. These diets may sometimes achieve quick results, but the weight loss is temporary and will be regained the moment you begin to eat in your normal pattern. Understand and study carefully the basic information in this chapter before embarking on a weight loss or gain program.

To determine the ideal proportions for your figure type, start by asking yourself a few questions. First, what is your bone structure? Do you have a small, medium, or large frame? You may tend to look around for someone with the perfect figure. That particular person may have an entirely different bone structure from yours. Consequently, determining that you want to look just like her is simply not realistic.

Second, consider age and activity level. Many people move quickly and are able to burn more energy or calories than others. You may know people who eat all they want and never gain a pound. If your manner is such that you move in a deliberate, relaxed pace, it will be necessary for you to compensate by eating fewer calories per day.

Third, carefully study your eating habits. When do you eat the most? Do you eat because of nervousness or happiness? Do you eat while watching television or studying?

Finally, how much are you willing to sacrifice to attain your ideal figure proportion goal? Reapportioning your figure means not only careful diet planning but also vigorous exercising. The attractive figure has correct proportions *and* firm muscle tone. But no matter how much you exercise, desired results will not be gained without calorie control. In this chapter, diet and exercise will be discussed, beginning by determining your figure type.

DETERMINING YOUR FIGURE TYPE

Begin your trimming program by consulting your physician. If you are overweight fifteen pounds or more, this is essential. It is always sound advice to consult your doctor before embarking on *any* strenuous weight loss or exercise program.

How do you know if you are overweight? Your tape measure can be your valuable friend and guide. Ideal weight cannot be determined without first determining your bone structure. To do this, measure your wrist just *below* the bone, holding the tape snugly. Record on your Personal Analysis Chart, Chart 2, to the nearest one-quarter inch, your wrist size. To interpret this measurement, refer to Table 2 which indicates small, medium, and large body structures.

TABLE 2

Determining body frame (by wrist measurements)

	Wrist Measurement[1]		Height		
	Inches	Feet	Inches	Feet	Inches
SMALL	5½ or less	5	2		or under
	6 or less	5	3 to	5	4
	6¼ or less	5	5 to	5	11
MEDIUM	5½ to 5¾	5	2		or under
	6 to 6¼	5	3 to	5	4
	6¼ to 6½	5	5 to	5	11
LARGE	5¾ or more	5	2		or under
	6¼ or more	5	3 to	5	4
	6½ or more	5	5 to	5	11

[1] *To determine frame, measure your wrist just below the bone to the nearest ¼ inch.*

CHART 2

Personal Analysis Chart

Name _____ Age _____

Height _____ Weight _____ Body Frame _____

Bust _____ Waist _____ Hip _____

Thigh _____ Calf _____ Ankle _____

Upper Arm _____ Abdomen _____ Wrist _____

Calories allowed per day _____

Calories eaten per day (Count every bite) _____

Most calories eaten _____ Morning _____ Between Meals _____ Night

Reason for eating _____ Boredom _____ Habit _____ Nervousness

_____ Celebration _____ Depression

Proposed goal	Increase	Decrease
Weight	_____	_____
Bust	_____	_____
Waist	_____	_____
Hip	_____	_____
Thigh	_____	_____
Calves	_____	_____
Abdomen	_____	_____
Upper Arm	_____	_____

Second, you will need to know your correct height. This measurement is taken by standing erect, in stocking feet, and holding the chin level. Give yourself the benefit of every quarter inch. You may be surprised that you have grown since your last measurement. Now, refer to Table 3, showing the ideal weight for your height and body structure.

Continue to record your vital statistics on the Personal Analysis Chart, Chart 2, by measuring the bust (over the fullest part), waist and hip (seven inches below natural waistline; however, this is not always the fullest part—be very critical in measuring).

Record next the thigh, calf, and ankle. The ankle measurement, unlike the wrist, is taken just *above* the ankle bone. Do not overlook the upper arm measurement. This is often where a person first tends to become flabby and show age.

For many years the rule of thumb has been a waist measurement ten inches smaller than the bust and hips: thirty-six, twenty-six, thirty-six. Because of the relaxed styles in dress waistlines for many years, the waistline has slipped drastically, up to three inches in some cases. Has yours? If not, you are luckier than most.

How do you measure up to the ideal proportions shown in Table 4? Do you fall within the boundaries in each scale? If so, consider yourself fortunate. At this point a few comments are in

TABLE 3

Normal weights for women[1]

Height		Small Frame	Medium Frame	Large Frame
Feet	Inches	Pounds	Pounds	Pounds
4	11	96-103	102-110	109-119
5	0	97-105	104-112	111-121
5	1	99-107	106-114	113-123
5	2	102-110	109-117	116-127
5	3	105-113	112-120	119-130
5	4	108-117	116-124	123-134
5	5	111-120	119-127	125-137
5	6	115-124	122-132	130-142
5	7	118-128	126-136	134-146
5	8	121-131	129-139	137-150
5	9	125-135	133-143	141-154
5	10	128-139	137-147	144-158
5	11	131-142	140-150	147-161

[1] *These tables have been worked out from numerous medical insurance studies. They represent average desirable weights by health standards. However, remember that individuals vary, as does weight distribution, and these figures must be adjusted to your individual requirements—the weight at which you look and feel best. (These are weights in pounds, without clothing, according to height and frame.)*

TABLE 4

Normal modern measurements[1]

Height		Neck	Bust	Upper Arm	Wrist	Waist	Abdomen	Hips	Thigh	Calf	Ankle
Feet	Inches	Inches	Inches	Inches	Inches	Inches	Inches	Inches	Inches	Inches	Inches
4	11	11½	31½	9	5	21	27	31½	18¼	11¼	7
5	0	11½	32	9¼	5¼	21½	27½	32	18½	11½	7¼
5	1	11¾	32½	9½	5½	22	28	32½	19	11¾	7½
5	2	12	33	9¾	5¾	22½	28½	33	19¼	12	7¾
5	3	12¼	33½	10	5¾	23	29	33¼	19½	12¼	8
5	4	12½	34	10¼	6	23½	29½	33½	20	12½	8¼
5	5	12½	34½	10½	6¼	24	30	34	20½	12¾	8½
5	6	12¾	35	10½	6½	24½	30½	34½	20¾	13	8¾
5	7	13	36	11	6½	25	31	35	21	13¼	8¾
5	8	13¼	36½	11	6½	25½	31½	35½	21¼	13½	8¾
5	9	13½	37	11	6½	26	32	36	21½	13½	8¾
5	10	13¾	37½	11¼	6¾	26½	32½	36½	21¾	13¾	8¾
5	11	13⅞	38	11½	6¾	27	32¾	37	22	13⅞	8¾
6	0	14	38½	11¾	6¾	27½	33	37½	22¼	14	9

[1] *These are measurements that have been worked out from a number of authoritative sources and modified to fit today's standards of beauty, which are somewhat different than those of a few years ago. The modern trend is toward the slender figure with curves in the right places.*

order about the person who is slightly underweight and therefore is slightly below the scale of measurements illustrated. Doctors have proven that people who are underweight tend to have more vitality and enjoy better health. Fashion designers have been designing clothes with you in mind! Do not worry about the charts, just think of the thousands of women who would gladly exchange your figure problem for theirs!

CALORIES COUNT

More than likely, you have not considered the fact that "you, too, will be thirty." You may not be aware of the fact that for every year between ages eighteen and twenty-five you may add one pound to the weight shown in Table 8. However, do not exceed by seven pounds the weight shown. Your weight becomes stabilized at age twenty-five. Do you find that your weight corresponds to the given chart if you add until the age forty?!!! If so, no time to *waist!*

The next step will be to compute your daily intake of calories. Be scrupulously honest in counting your calories. This means every bite of candy, sip of cola, or crunch of peanut. You will find a pocket version calorie counter (available for about thirty cents at food and drug stores) a valuable help. Table 5 is a concise listing of what are called "trouble foods" that tend to add excess poundage because of their snack packaging or appeal to one's taste for sweets.

TABLE 5

Calorie chart

Item	Portion	Calories
Pancakes	1 portion	62
Hamburger bun	1 portion	85-130
Hot dog bun	1 portion	85-115
Candy bar (nuts)	2 oz.	271
Almond Joy	2 pieces	296
Hershey Bar		154
Lifesavers	1 piece	10
White mint	1 piece	6
M & M's	1 package—small	138
Popcorn	1 cup (no butter)	54
Cereals	1 cup	100-110
Cookies (cream filled)	1 piece	57
Nut brownie	1 piece	80
Vanilla wafer	1 piece	18
Crackers	1 piece	15-20
Pretzels	1 oz.	107
Corn chips	1 oz.	168
Potato chips	1 oz.	155
Butter	½ oz.	50
	1 teaspoon	100
Margarine	same as butter	
Cheese	1 oz.	113
Italian cheese	1 oz.	90
Cottage cheese	1 cup	215
Whipped cream	4 oz.	414
Eggs	1	70
Eggs (scrambled)	1	112
Steak (sirloin)	4 oz.	352
Pork chop	4 oz.	408
Veal cutlet	4 oz.	191
Liver	3 oz.	119
Chicken (roast)	3 oz.	100
Fish (flounder)	3½ oz.	79
Vegetables		
Green beans	3½ oz.	42
Green pepper	$\frac{1}{8}$ cup	4
Tomatoes (fresh)	3½ oz.	23
Fruit		
Apples	1 medium	65
Bananas	1 medium	80
Pears	1 small	70
Carbonated drinks	6 oz.	82
Diet drinks	6 oz.	6

Also listed are several snack foods high in protein and food value. The secret in developing good eating habits is to substitute low-calorie foods for high-caloried snacks. Remember the old saying, "A moment on the lips, a lifetime on the hips."

Perhaps another incentive to watch your eating habits is to paste pictures of obese people at danger points such as on the refrigerator door or inside the pantry. The positive approach would be to use pictures of trim people in bikini bathing suits in such spots and in the bathroom near the mirror. The saying, "Fat and happy," is another of the diet myths. Statistics prove that people who are fat often eat because they are unhappy.

Now that you have determined *what* you eat daily, strive to determine *why* you ate it. On your Personal Analysis Chart, a space is provided for recording daily intake of *all* calories with a margin for *why*. Some people eat to ease tension before an important exam, job interview, or special date. Others eat to celebrate a job promotion, at a special weekend party, or because of a sale purchase. You might eat because of boredom or as a method of occupying your hands while reading or watching television.

A helpful hint is to keep a package of gum readily available. Gum has very few calories, one to five per stick, and will give the stomach the sensation of eating a snack. It is also a means of relieving tension. It goes without saying that you must chew gum in private. Chewing gum in public is a breach of good manners and business etiquette.

Here is a handy calorie count guide:

GUIDE 4

Calorie Count Guide

The normally active person (over twenty) may consume fifteen calories a day per pound of body weight. Example: 120 pounds × 15 calories = 1800 calories per day.

One pound of body fat contains 3500 calories. Thus, to lose one pound per week, cut out 500 calories per day for one week. Example: one chocolate malt, one piece of pie with whipped cream topping, or two small chocolate candy bars.

**PERSONAL ACTIVITY LEVEL
OR "THE HARE AND THE TORTOISE"**

Your activity level determines to a great extent the amount of energy you consume daily and therefore the calories you burn. Do you prefer to walk or run? Do you walk to school or work instead of riding the bus or car? Do you climb stairs when an elevator is available? Do you participate in active sports, or do you prefer to be a spectator? Can you sit for hours reading a book or daydreaming, or do you jump up and down many times while studying or pursuing a hobby?

Metabolism, too, plays an important part in the way your body uses your food intake. Thyroid imbalance may affect the assimilation of your calories; however, more often poor eating habits or nervousness are the major causes of obesity.

The number of calories you can burn in a half-hour of different kinds of vigorous exercise are listed in the following chart.

Cycling	up to 585
Walking (fast)	up to 550
Roller skating	up to 685
Ice skating	up to 700
Dancing	up to 730
Golf (not riding in cart)	up to 565
Tennis	up to 805
Basketball	up to 805
Field hockey	up to 805
Swimming	up to 685
Rowing	up to 1300
Skiing (Snow)	up to 625
Skiing (Water)	up to 600

You can readily see from the chart that a person who participates actively in an exercise or recreation program has the opportunity to burn many more calories than the person who merely watches. The spectator will have to compensate for lack of exercise by controlling the daily caloric intake.

EATING HABITS

Statistics show that although our society today is affluent, people are undernourished. This is due in part to the availability of prepackaged and prepared foods, which may be satisfying to the appetite but contain little food value.

Do you know about vitamins and the part they play in maintaining a healthy body and sound mind? How often have you considered the protein value in the foods you eat daily? The seven most complete protein foods today, those loaded with nutrients but low in calories, are cheese, eggs, fish, meat (lean), chicken, skim milk, and wheat germ. Increased intake of protein (above the daily required amount) helps burn up fat at the rate of seventy-five to one hundred grams per day. Protein improves your reflexes, gives you more energy, promotes healthier skin, hair, and nails, and improves the posture. A midday or late afternoon slump may result as the level of blood sugar drops. For a quick lift to carry you through this slump, substitute protein for candy or other sugar products.

The use of vitamins can be helpful in achieving specific results. The increased intake of vitamin A aids in correcting dry skin problems and visual defects such as night blindness. Vitamin E assures normal body reproduction processes, a lack of which is related to infertility, muscular dystrophy, and other vascular abnormalities. A lack of niacin can result in depression, forgetfulness, suspicion, and instability. It is sometimes referred to as the "morale" vitamin. Vitamin D is a great aid to the oily skin victim and helps clear blemishes.

It is important to maintain a well-balanced diet to guard against such severe deficiencies. If your eating habits are poor, supplement your diet with a daily multiple vitamin. Most women are iron deficient, and we suggested that you consider a vitamin high in iron content.

DAILY DIET PLAN

Plan ahead. Educate yourself so that you are aware of the calorie count of every bite you place in your mouth. It is easier to count calories if you have a friend to help. You might adopt the motto, "We diet quiet," and see how long it takes for your friends to notice the change.

Be sure to plan several small meals a day instead of three large ones. Drink all the diet drink your stomach will hold before each meal, but no water or beverage with your meal. This cuts down your appetite.

Save your low calorie dessert until you are studying or watching TV later in the evening. Bedtime snacks often add many useless calories to your quota. In exercising a *sensible* diet plan, try to cut down on desserts without eliminating them completely. Cutting them out completely will result in an intense craving for sweets that destroys previous progress in weight reduction.

Cut out the salt-shake habit. Do not add additional salt to food after it has been prepared. Keep an ample supply of low calorie foods in your pantry and refrigerator. It may be necessary to educate your mother if your family has a meal plan consisting of rich casseroles, fried foods, vegetables in sauces, and heavy desserts. More important is to educate yourself so that you can choose the lowest calorie menu whether it is in the school cafeteria, the luncheon snack bar, or an elegant restaurant for dinner.

TRYING TO GAIN WEIGHT

As hard as it may seem for the generally overweight or slightly overweight person, there are a number of people today who try every conceivable type of food and food supplement to gain weight. It generally results in failure because the basic nature of such persons is to expend much more energy accomplishing their daily routine than the slower moving, obese person does. It is hard to dispel the theory that because you are thin you are not strong!

The following suggestions can help you gain weight. You want this weight to be firm—not fat! If your appetite is especially particular, take time to prepare your meals so that they appear appetizing as well as being nutritionally wholesome.

Eat slowly, and try to lie down for a short nap or rest after each meal. Slowing down your rate of metabolism is very difficult. Use food supplements as bedtime snacks. This will assure the maximum benefit for your intake. Do not skip meals. Be sure that you supplement your diet with vitamins and iron-enriched foods. This can help to increase your appetite. You will gradually train yourself to eat more each day if you increase your nutritious foods, if you eat more slowly, and if you give yourself time to digest each bite. Cut down on snacking. Do not smoke. Smoking curbs the appetite.

If you are extremely nervous, consult your physician. He may suggest a mild medication to help you combat this problem. It is also important not to let yourself be intimidated by suggestions that you try to gain weight or that you look too thin. This will only complicate your problem and cause you to worry needlessly, thus further affecting your appetite.

EXERCISE

Motivation plays the biggest part in developing a sound daily exercise program. Forms of motivation are varied, and the key to success is in choosing the one most applicable to you and your figure needs. You must prepare yourself psychologically to initiate this program. The inability to fit into last year's favorite knit dress or cocktail suit, the challenge of fitting into a dress one size smaller, or a longing for a cute new tennis outfit that accentuates your not-so-slim hipline may do it.

Set your goals and go about achieving them one day at a time. You will find that you actually feel better and are more mentally alert when you exercise daily. There are many excellent exercise programs available to follow, but the most effective one is the one you do at least five times per week. It is suggested that you pick a certain time of day to exercise and use it consistently. Exercise slowly and deliberately to get the most out of it. Exercising at the same time of day will help you develop it into a *habit* as part of your daily routine.

TIP-TO-TOE ANALYSIS

Now is a good time to pull out the tape measure again and take another careful look at your particular problem areas. It is advisable to incorporate circulatory exercises into your program. These aid in the stimulation of blood flow and strengthen the heart and lung muscles. Such exercises also increase the flow of blood to the brain and will enable you to think more clearly and perform your job more efficiently.

Begin your exercise program with the face. Understand that tension, lack of sleep, and climate play important parts in the deterioration of facial muscles. It is important to remember a few simple exercises for the face.

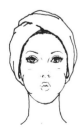

That Fabulous Face
1. Exaggerate vowel sounds (A, E, I, O, U) (Repeat this series ten times to relax muscles.)
2. Blow out the cheeks, release the breath slowly to the count of ten, build up the count to twenty. (See Figure 62.) This exercise eases lines on either side of the nose and mouth.

FIGURE 62.

139

3. Exaggerate *wh* sound: *wh*at, *wh*ere, *wh*y, *wh*en, (Do the series ten times beginning slowly, then faster with each series of repetition.)

4. Hold your head erect; spank yourself firmly under the chin with the back of the hands, alternately using an upward and outward motion. This exercise firms the throat muscles.

5. Vibrate the entire face and neck with your fingertips by gently patting in a fluttery, circular motion.

Continue your exercise program by moving on to the neck area.

The Neck: As Graceful as a Swan—Or Is It?

1. Sitting erect, chest lifted, head up, tense the throat muscles and slowly turn your head until the chin is pointed over your right shoulder. Raise and lower the chin to the shoulder five times; then turn your head in the other direction and raise and lower chin to the left shoulder five times.

2. Tip your head straight back, looking directly at the ceiling; chew slowly, opening your mouth wide, pulling up strongly with the lower jaw muscles to close your mouth. Try this ten times, working up to twenty.

3. Neck circling: Sitting or standing, *slowly* drop the head to the right, down in front, to the left, and backward, making a complete circle. This is a good exercise to relieve tension. (See Figure 63).

4. Dowager's hump: Stand straight with your mouth open, drop the head forward and backward ten times. Drop it as far as possible each way so that you feel the muscles pull. Keep your mouth open.

To make neck and facial exercising more effective, clean the face and neck thoroughly and apply a face cream to the entire area

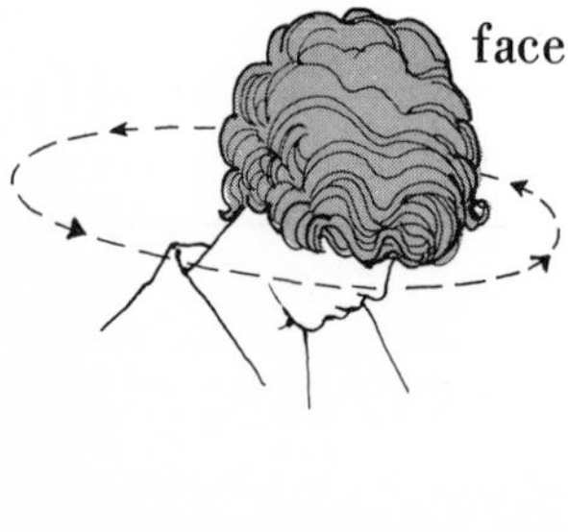

FIGURE 63.
Neck circling.

and a rich lubricating cream, such as a throat cream, to the neck area before exercising. This will make the skin more supple and will increase the benefit of the various suggested exercises.

Following are arm and shoulder exercise suggestions:

Ample Arm Attempts

1. Arm rotations: Sit or stand with your arms outstretched to shoulder level. Circle the arms ten times in a clockwise direction. Relax and repeat ten times in a counterclockwise direction. Start with small circles and progress to large circles (Figure 64).

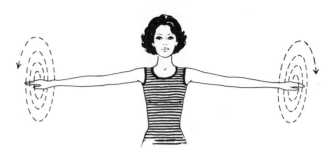

FIGURE 64.

2. Stand with your arms outstretched at shoulder level, palms down; swing your arms forward and cross them in front, forming an "X." Hold the crossed position for a few seconds until you feel it pull, and then relax. Repeat ten times.

3. Rowing: Sit or stand with your elbows bent and held out at shoulder level with your hands in front of your chest. Swing the elbows back as far as possible ten to twenty times in rapid succession.

4. Chest lift: Lie flat on your stomach with your arms clasped behind your neck, elbows out. Draw your shoulders together and raise your chest and head off the floor. Relax, and repeat several times.

5. Stand with your feet slightly apart, your arms straight down at your sides. Raise your arms up and over your head until they cross. For more effect and to help increase the bustline, hold small books in each hand and do this exercise ten to twenty times.

In toning the body, do not neglect the back area. The following exercises firm these muscles and help ease tension as well.

Beautiful Back

1. Lie on your back with your arms above your head and your knees bent. Move one knee as far as you can toward your chest, and simultaneously straighten out the other leg. Return to the original position with both knees bent and repeat the movements, changing legs. Relax, and repeat ten times.

2. Sit on a straight chair. Let your body drop forward until your head is down between your knees. Pull your body back up into an upright position as you tighten your abdominal muscles. Relax, and repeat the exercise six times (Figure 65).

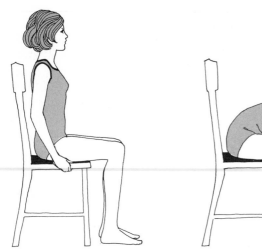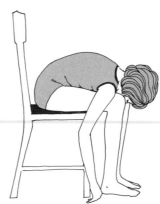

FIGURE 65.
The back builder.

3. Lie on the floor and relax with your arms above your head and your knees bent. Now tighten the muscles of your lower abdomen and your buttocks simultaneously in order to flatten your back against the floor. Hold the position for ten counts. Relax, and repeat the exercise. This is excellent to correct a swayback or slightly curved spine.

The midriff often slacks and results in a midriff bulge. These specific exercises help correct this situation.

Midriff Minimizers

1. The twist: Stand with your feet about eighteen inches apart, perfect posture, arms outstretched to the side at shoulder level. Swing the arms and upper part of the torso to the left as far as possible without moving the hips. Swing the arms and upper body back as far as possible to the right, keeping the hips stationary. Repeat ten times to each side. (See Figure 66.)

2. Waist stretch: Stand straight with good posture, legs apart, right arm up. Bend sidewise, slide the left arm and hand down along the side of the left thigh and leg as far as you can. Repeat with the right arm. Perform this exercise several times on each side, slowly, without jerking. (Warm up first.) Build up to ten times.

3. Waist-hip roll: Lie on the floor, arms outstretched to the side, knees bent and brought up to the bustline. Tense the stomach muscles and roll the knees first to the right side, touching the floor, and then to the left side, touching the floor. Start out at ten and gradually work up to thirty or forty times. This is fun and relaxing if you pick a soft spot such as a carpet or rug, but it is more effective if it is done on a hard surface.

Stomach muscles relax with age. A regular series of tummy exercises will control this condition.

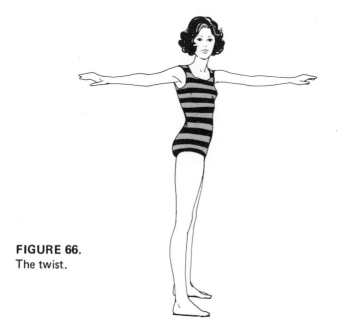

FIGURE 66.
The twist.

Tummy Tightener

The plain old-fashioned sit-up: Lie on your back with your hands clasped behind your head and your knees bent with your feet near your hips. Bring your head and shoulders forward until your right elbow touches your left knee. Return to the starting position, then touch the left elbow to the right knee. Exercise five times and gradually add a few each day, working up to twenty-five.

Hips cause many people concern. *Controlling* the hip proportions by exercise is easier than reducing the hip size.

Hip Helpers

1. Fanny walk: Sit on the floor, back straight, arms stretched out in front, legs stretched out. In little "hitching" movements, walk across the floor from one end of the room to the other. Then, without turning, bump backward to the starting position. Be sure the movement is not a sliding one. There must be a definite lift of the body each time, and the thigh should be dropped to the floor with a sharp slap. This is a good massage for troublesome hip and pone contour. Pone is the deposit of fatty tissue that builds up and causes a bulge at the hip joint.

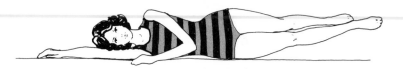

FIGURE 67.
Scissors.

2. Scissors: Lie on one side with one arm under the head and the other in front to use as a support. The legs should be held straight with the knees rigid. Move the legs back and forth in quick, vigorous strides, as in opening and closing scissors. Keep the legs elevated and above the floor. Start on the right side and work back and forth twenty-five times. Turn over to the left side and do another twenty-five vigorous crosses. (See Figure 67.)

Trim legs and thighs are most attractive. Exercise provides a graceful curve. Follow these suggestions.

Lovelier Legs—and Thighs

1. Standing hold the back of a chair with one hand. Raise the right leg out to the side as high as you can. Hold it there a moment; then *from that point*, kick higher. Do not make the mistake of dropping the leg even a few inches for a second kick—you will never get the right pull on that muscle. The second kick must come from that out-stretched position that seems as high as you were able to raise the leg in the first movement. Repeat this ten times, then kick-hold-kick with the left leg ten times. Alternate legs. This helps keep the legs more flexible and does away with some of that bulge or pone on the upper outer thigh.

2. Ballet bar kick: Stand with your hand on a chair or waist-high bar. Kick one leg forward as far as it will stretch, keeping the stomach muscles tight. Then swing the leg backward as far as you can; also keep all your muscles tight and your toes pointed. Do this ten times, working up to twenty, with each leg.

3. Bicycle run: Lie on your back, hands supporting the hips at your waistline. Raise the feet and hips into the air and pedal the legs vigorously as though you were riding a bicycle. Do this twenty times, rest a minute, and repeat another twenty times. (See Figure 68.)

Ankles must not be neglected. These exercises are simple and may be done with little effort, but produce noticeable results.

Ankles Aweigh

1. Pedaling: Alternately rise up on the toe of one foot, ankle

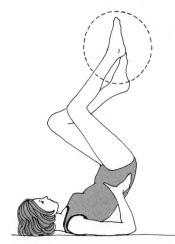

FIGURE 68.
Bicycle run.

extended, while keeping the heel of the other foot on the floor. Start gently, softly, slowly, gradually increasing the tempo until you are running in place.

2. Skywriting: Lie on your back, knees bent. Cross the right leg over the left, and use the big toe to write your name in the air. Repeat with the left foot. A good word to practice with is: *supercalifragelisticexpealidotious*.

3. Ankles around: Sit on a chair with the right leg crossed over the left and rotate the right ankle clockwise ten times, then counterclockwise ten times. Reverse the position—the left leg over the right, and repeat the series. (See Figure 69.)

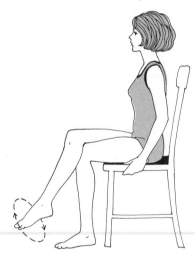

FIGURE 69.
Ankles around.

Exercises for the feet greatly help reduce fatigue. A series of these exercises followed by a hot foot bath produces immediate relief of foot fatigue.

Featuring the Feet

1. Sit on a chair or low stool with one foot placed on the floor. (Toe in, with weight on the outer border, greater toe touching the floor.) Pick up small objects with the toes of the other foot and place them on the knee of the stationary leg, with the thigh of the working leg rotated outward and the knee as low as possible. Repeat, using the other foot. Continue to repeat the exercise until the feet tingle with increased circulation.

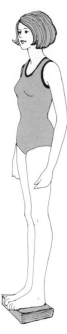

2. Stand on the edge of a large telephone book or mat, with the toes reaching over the edge; grip the edge of the book or mat with the toes while the weight is thrown onto the center of the feet. Try to lift the edge of the book off the floor (Figure 70).

3. Grasp a pencil under the toes of one foot, with the writing end beyond the little toe, and write with large strokes. Do the same with the other foot.

Pretty hands are immediately noticeable to a casual admirer. Exercise helps keep hands supple and increases circulation.

Happy Hands

1. Relax the fingers with elbows bent, fling and shake the hands rapidly.

2. Sit or stand with arms to the sides, holding a page of newspaper in each hand. Start at one corner of the page, and curl and uncurl the fingers, crumpling the paper until the entire page is in the hand. (See Figure 71.)

3. Soak your hands in warm oil—three tablespoons of baby oil or olive oil. While your hands are warm and moist, work the skin of the fingers and hand toward the wrist as though you were putting on gloves. Massage and stimulate each finger separately, starting with the right hand. Then repeat the motions with left hand. When the "gloves are on," gently dry your hands, always working the skin from the tips of the fingers toward the wrist bone. This should be done also when applying lotion or cream to hands to minimize the veins, which sometimes become prominent.

FIGURE 70.

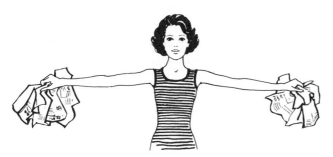

FIGURE 71.
Helping hands.

We cannot complete this chapter without a bit of explanation about circulatory exercises. There are many methods such as jogging. *Key to Fitness at Any Age—The New Aerobics*[1] is an excellent book. The exercises featured in *Adult Physical Fitness*[2] prepared by the President's Council on Physical Fitness for Men and Women may be used. Jumping rope for the person who for one reason or another chooses an on-the-premises exercise is also good. Most physicians recommend these forms of exercise as the most effective to combat heart disease. Isometric exercises play an important part in maintaining muscle tone once you have gotten your body back into shape. The following are suggestions for exercises that can be done while sitting at your desk, riding in the car, or lying in bed.

Circulatory Suggestions

1. Tummy: Tense the stomach muscles, inhaling sharply and holding to the count of ten; exhale and count to ten. Repeat this as many times as possible. This will work inches off your waistline if it is done regularly.

2. Ankle slimmer: Sit at a desk and extend your legs forward. With the toes pointed, very quickly cross and uncross your legs at the ankles until blood circulation increases and your legs begin to tingle.

3. Face exercise: Contort your face in a spectrum of expressions—exaggerate laughing, frowning, eating sour foods, blowing bubbles, sucking through a straw, and so on. This is to be done in privacy or you will draw sidelong glances from students and coworkers.

4. Sit tall, with your back firmly against the back of your chair; try to push your stomach muscles through the back of the chair.

5. When bending, reaching, sitting, or lying on your back in bed, simultaneously tense and tuck in all the body muscles you can. Hold for a count of ten and repeat it. It is amazing what pinching in the buttocks and tightening the stomach muscles will do. It will soon become an automatic

[1]Kenneth H. Cooper, *Key to Fitness at Any Age—The New Aerobics* (New York: M. Evans and Co., 1970).

[2] President's Council on Physical Fitness for Men and Women, *Adult Physical Fitness* (Washington, D.C.: Superintendent of Documents; Government Printing Office).

habit and not only will you look better but your posture will improve as well.

The information presented in this chapter concerning exercise and diet will benefit you little if you develop an "on again, off again" attitude. Results will be accomplished by changing your present lifestyle and developing sounder ideas regarding the importance of physical fitness in your daily life. Experiment with the suggested exercises listed in this chapter, and adopt a set basic to your figure needs and desires. Pursue your goal faithfully—one day at a time—and you will soon be in trim with the times.

ENRICHMENT ACTIVITIES

1. Compile a cookbook of diet recipes. Exchange helpful hints with classmates on ways to prepare low calorie and tasty foods.

2. Study the vitamin and protein value of foods. Know how to achieve significant results by introducing extra amounts of vitamins and proteins into your daily diet.

3. Prepare a cartoon clipping file pertaining to weight control— poems, sayings, and illustrations. Find both positive and negative examples.

4. Stand in front of a mirror; draw an imaginary line down the center. List assets on one side, liabilities on the other. Total. Do your liabilities outweigh your assets? If so, get to work. Be fair. Consider all points: hair, skin, figure, and so on.

5. Start a file of periodicals, newspaper articles, technical journals, and pamphlets about physical fitness, and sound mental behavior patterns, diet, and exercise.

6. Purchase a thirty-cent calorie counter. Study until you can determine the approximate value of all the foods you eat each day and thus cut down on needless caloric intake. This will be fun as well as surprising in some cases.

7. Prepare a chart illustrating a simple one-thousand-calorie-per-day diet for one week. Be sure to keep your diet nutritionally balanced.

necessities and such...
for women only

The vibrant woman in today's society, whether she is a career or college girl, married or single, is constantly looking for new challenges to expand her mind as well as new methods and modes of dress and makeup to enhance her beauty. She wants to project an independent contemporary image that proves to the world that she is not only aware of its happenings but also a vital contributor to them.

This chapter deals with some very delicate subjects of utmost importance to today's woman. However, all but the most fastidious women may take these subjects for granted. They are simply reminders of the many hygienic details that go into making the meticulous, contemporary female.

Much information is available today in books, magazines, and the news media on keeping in good physical shape and being well-groomed from tip to toe. The vibrant woman knows there is no excuse for anything less than an immaculate, neat appearance at all times.

How does she achieve this appearance? In addition to adequate rest, exercise, proper diet, and regular medical checkups, today's woman has learned that being well-groomed is the result of nothing more than establishing good grooming habits.

Cicero said, "Habit is almost a second nature," but we are never too old to develop new habits. Some career women perform a beauty routine each evening they are at home. For example, one evening the career girl may shampoo her hair and possibly give herself a manicure while she is under the dryer. A second evening she may give herself a pedicure (Chapter Six). On a third evening she may remove superfluous hair from her legs, face, and underarms. A college girl, on the other hand, with studies on most weekday evenings, may prefer to do all of her beauty chores on one weekend afternoon or free evening. It doesn't matter when these chores are done—the important thing is that they are done regularly and *before* the need becomes obvious.

THE TRANQUIL BATH

The daily bathing habit was established for most of us when we were infants, so the most essential grooming chore is already part of our daily schedule. However, are you allowing yourself the real luxury of a totally tranquilizing, unrushed bath each day? Do you remember, as a child, playing for hours in a tub of warm, bubbly water? How refreshing it was! As you grew older and demands began to be made upon your time, perhaps bathing became only another job to be completed—another task to be rushed through.

For the busy college and career girl, the thought of a fifteen-minute bath may seem like an eternity. After the hectic pace of a rushed day at the office or on campus, you may feel you cannot afford the time. This is all the more reason you need this luxury. The

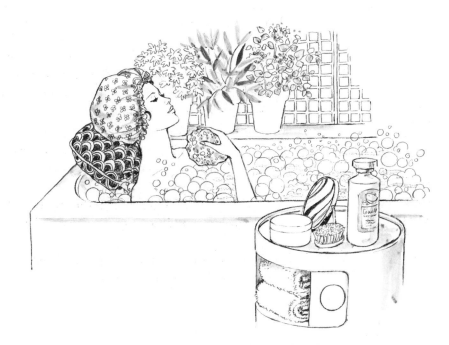

FIGURE 72.

quick shower you take before you leave home in the mornings helps you get started and refreshed, but it does not give you the tranquilizing effect that sitting in a warm tub of water and completely unwinding at the end of a busy day does. The tranquilizing bath helps relax every muscle and calm every nerve in your body while washing away the grime and dirt that today's pollution leaves on you (Figure 72).

The time of day you set aside for your bath depends entirely upon your particular lifestyle. The college girl may find the early evening her best time to bathe. Then she will be refreshed to study or go out. The career woman, particularly if she has a family, may find that her best time is after the children are in bed and before she retires for the evening. Below are some hints that will help make your tranquilizing bath the highlight of your day:

1. Make sure the tub is thoroughly clean and has been disinfected, particularly if it is a dormitory or hotel tub, which could harbor bacteria of athlete's foot or other infections.

2. Fill the tub about three-quarters full of warm water. Add bath oil, crystals, bubbles, or whatever you prefer. Plain baby oil is an inexpensive but effective bath oil. Recipe for frazzled nerves: Mix, in a piece of cheesecloth, a handful each of rosemary, thyme, dried mint, a half handful of lavender leaves, one orange peel, one lemon peel, and one tablespoon of dried lemon. Tie the cheesecloth securely and toss it into an empty tub; fill the tub with hot water. Let the solution steep for ten minutes, climb in, and find out how the heavenly scent will soothe your nerves.

3. Have your toilet articles—towels, cloth, nightgown, robe, or other clothing—within easy reach.

4. Don your shower cap, and cream your neck and face.

5. Stretch out in the warm water. Let every muscle relax. You may wish to put a rolled towel under your neck as a pillow.

6. Do some exercises while your body is buoyant. In this weightless condition, exercises are easy to do and very beneficial.

7. While soaping and washing your body, also "wash" your mind of every care and worry.

8. Rinse off or use a lukewarm, or even cool, shower if you prefer.

9. Step out of the tub and briskly dry yourself. Push back the cuticles on your toes and fingers with the towel, and rub your heels, elbows, and feet to loosen dead skin.

10. Cream your body with moisturizing lotion if you have dry skin, or dust yourself with your favorite bath powder. Apply deodorant and cologne or perfume.

You will feel like a new person! The energy you now have will more than make up for the fifteen minutes you may have spent bathing.

FRAGRANCE

There is nothing more feminine than the smell of a perfumed woman. Since before Cleopatra, females have been using fragrances of one kind or another. Fragrance can have a tantalizing effect on people. They are no longer limited only to women—many men use cologne regularly.

Many types of fragrances are available today:

Perfume has the highest percentage of concentrated oils. It should be applied sparingly because it is so strong. Apply it strategically: at the pulse points on wrists and throat, behind the knees, and between the breasts. Even though perfume is more expensive than cologne or toilet water, it is more economical in the long run because you use less of it.

Toilet water and cologne are diluted forms of perfume. These can be applied more generously than perfume. They can also be sprayed from an atomizer. Some women prefer cologne because of its lighter fragrance. Madame Jacqueline Goddet, a Parisian who is active in the fragrance industry, recommends that you spray your linen closets with toilet water. She also recommends spraying the air conditioning vents and putting a drop of perfume on the light bulbs so that when the lights are turned on, the entire room will be lightly scented.

Bath bubbles, bath gels, and *bath oils* are various forms of scented beauty and bath aids that soften the water as well as the skin.

Sachets and *bath powders* also contain scents. A satin-covered pouch of sachet slipped between lingerie in your dresser drawer will leave a delicious fragrance.

Moisturizers are creamy liquids to be applied to your body after your bath. These are particularly good for dry skin. Some moisturizers and bath powders contain the same fragrances as colognes.

Fragrance "Dos"

1. DO apply fragrance daily after your bath and shower and as often as needed during the day.
2. DO buy perfume in small sizes so that it will not lose its potency before you have finished the bottle.
3. DO carry a small atomizer in your purse for fresh applications.
4. DO wear less perfume in summer months because heat tends to intensify fragrance.

Fragrance "Don'ts"

1. DON'T spray perfume directly on clothing because it can stain.
2. DON'T substitute perfume for a bath or to camouflage body odor.
3. DON'T place perfume in sunlight because it loses its strength more rapidly.
4. DON'T use too much fragrance—it is better to be conservative than offensive.

Your Selection of Perfume. There are hundreds of different scents on the market today. It is estimated that some ten to thirty thousand scents can be identified—that is, if you have what is known in the fragrance industry as a "successful nose." With so many different scents available, selecting the right one can become a difficult task. Just as a certain shade of lipstick may appear one color on your friend and an entirely different color on you, so it is with the odor of perfume. The skin and body chemistry of each person reacts differently; therefore, a fragrance that smells divine on one person may go completely sour on another.

Select your perfume with great care, just as you would your wardrobe or a fine piece of furniture or art. Because too many scents can confuse the inexperienced nose, never dab on more than three scents at any one time while trying to make your selection. Your first clue that you have selected the right fragrance is when a special someone tells you he likes the way you smell.

Some women change perfumes as frequently as hairstyles. Other women would rather fight than switch, and their fragrance soon becomes their "trademark."

YOUR PERSONAL NEEDS

The tranquilizing bath and the sweet, sweet smell of perfume would all be for naught were it not for the mighty odor stoppers available today. Deodorants and antiperspirants are a regular part of the grooming and feminine hygiene of today's fastidious woman. In a survey made of businessmen and women, a small percentage indicated that body odor was still a definite problem among a few women working in their offices or places of business. Because of the delicacy of getting the point across to the offender without being brazen, some were fired without being told the real reason for their dismissals.

In today's sophisticated society, with one deodorant commercial after another on television, it is inexcusable for any mature person to not use a deodorant. Because of their tremendous effectiveness, deodorants are probably the most economical personal commodity available on the market today.

Glands. There are two types of glands that produce perspiration. The *apocrine* glands are located under the arms, and the *eccrine* glands are located all over the body. The eccrine glands produce perspiration, but it is odorless. Perspiration from the apocrine glands contains certain acids that bacteria feed on. When this perspiration is decomposed by bacteria, an underarm odor is produced. The perspiration from the eccrine glands does *not* feed the bacteria, which is why there is no odor. If perspiration from the eccrine glands is kept enclosed for long periods of time, in close areas such as shoes, an odor can form. This odor is not caused by acids in the perspiration but by bacteria decomposing dead skin on the feet. It takes very little emotion or stress to activate the underarm apocrine glands. These facts may help you determine which type of deodorant to use and how often to use it.

How Often? Experts say there are very few cases of underarm odor that cannot be controlled with an effective deodorant applied at least once a day and a thorough bath every twenty-four hours. Some deodorant specialists believe you should apply deodorant fifteen minutes or so after your bath. By then the pores will have had time to close. If you are a college girl and under unusual stress, such as before an examination; or if you are a career woman and under stress because of a new job, deodorant should be applied more often. Some women apply deodorant after bathing at night and again in the morning. You are the best judge of how often to apply it, but if you are in doubt, use it more often.

Deodorant or Antiperspirant? Since all deodorants reduce perspiration, how do you decide which one to use? If you perspire a great deal, then an antiperspirant will be more effective for you.

Deodorants come in many forms: liquids, creams, roll-ons, sprays, and on small pads. The only way to discover the deodorant for your particular needs is to try several until you find the one that works most effectively for you.

Many people who perspire profusely wear dress shields that protect their clothing from perspiration stains. It is also a good idea to carry a small bottle of antiperspirant in your purse and excuse yourself for a fresh application when you begin to perspire.

Feminine Hygiene Deodorant Sprays. It is important to be especially conscientious about hygiene, bathing, and deodorant use during your menstrual period. There are many powders and sprays made especially for women. These deodorants are made to spray or powder on the external vaginal area. For convenience, most of these can be sprayed while the bottle is in either an upright or an inverted position. The powders may be used on sanitary pads to destroy the odor caused by menstrual discharge. These feminine deodorants should be used as often as necessary but especially during the monthly period. Some women are allergic to certain sprays and powders, so it may be wise to test the deodorant on a small portion of your skin before using it lavishly.

Sanitary Napkins and Tampons. Women who have an unusually heavy flow find that using sanitary napkins decreases the chance of a feminine accident. However, when napkins are used, it is essential to change them frequently. The feminine deodorant should be used at each change. The chance of an offensive odor is greater when you use a napkin because the discharge is outside the body and absorbed into the napkin. This is another reason for frequent changings. Some women find that using sanitary napkins on their heavy flow days and tampons on their beginning and waning days is more comfortable.

Tampons are worn internally, and unless your flow is heavy, the chance of odor is not quite as great as with the napkin. A great many women today prefer the comfort and freedom the tampon allows. Many girls, however, prefer to use the napkin until they marry. If you have a question about using the tampon, check with your gynecologist.

Excessive Hair. There is nothing so unattractive as superfluous hair on the face, arms, legs, and underarms. The meticulous woman always removes the hair before the need for it becomes apparent. There are many methods of hair removal.

1. *Razors.* Electric and safety razors are the most common method for removing hair from legs and underarms. Electric razors are quick and clean but do not give as close a shave as the old-fashioned safety razor.

2. *Bleaching and waxing.* Dark hair of fine texture may be bleached rather than removed from the face and arms. However, if the hair is thick and dark, it should be removed with a wax or gentle cream depilatory.

3. *Depilatory.* When you use a depilatory for the first time, be sure to test a small area inside your arm to be sure that your skin is not sensitive to it. This is particularly important for facial depilatories. If your skin in the test area becomes red and begins to itch, you are probably allergic to the depilatory. Be sure to follow the timing instructions precisely.

4. *Tweezers.* Tweezers are excellent for removing stray hairs under the eyebrow (never above brows). You may temporarily remove long, stiff hairs that suddenly appear on your face by tweezing them in a good light with a magnifying mirror. Get in the habit of looking for these little hairs daily. If they persist, you may want to consider electrolysis.

5. *Electrolysis.* If depilatories do not remove the hair effectively, you may wish to have it removed by electrolysis. This is a method whereby an electric needle is used to destroy the hair follicle. This method may be used on

the legs and other parts of the body as well as on the face. It is the most expensive but the most permanent method of hair removal. Ask your dermatologist or your family doctor to recommend an ethical electrologist. Careless and unskillful operators could permanently damage your skin.

FOR LIFE'S SAKE

Physical and Dental Checkups. You cannot be a vibrant woman unless you are a live one! Because both dental and physical hygiene are essential to being healthy and well-groomed, the vibrant woman realizes that regular medical checkups should be as much a part of her routine as regular skin and hair care. The old saying, "An ounce of prevention is worth a pound of cure," is certainly true when it concerns your health and life. The importance of a yearly physical examination by your physician and dentist cannot be overstressed. If your physician does not routinely give them, ask for a chest x-ray, urinalysis, blood test, pelvic examination, breast examination, and Pap test.

Selecting a Physician. If you do not have a physician, you should select one with the greatest of care. Because you are a woman and gynecologists deal with functions and diseases peculiar to women, you should be extremely thoughtful in your selection of him or her. Throughout the years, there will be many questions you may want to ask, and being able to talk frankly and professionally is essential.

Cancer.[1] Surpassed only by heart disease, cancer is one of the leading causes of death in America today. Over three hundred and fifty thousand people die of this dread disease every year. Many of these are women. The three forms of cancer that cause the most deaths are: (1) breast cancer (occurring almost exclusively in women); (2) colon and rectum cancer; and (3) uterine cancer (occurring exclusively in women).

Uterine Cancer and The Pap Test. The American Cancer Society suggests that women have a yearly Pap test. This test can detect cancer of the uterus in its earliest stages. Many thousands of women die of uterine cancer every year, but if it is found in its early

[1]The information about cancer in this chapter was obtained from pamphlets supplied by the American Cancer Society.

stages, it is almost always curable. This painless and inexpensive Pap test can be done by your gynecologist or physician. The doctor removes a small amount of fluid from the mouth of the uterus. This fluid is then examined for cells that might be or become cancer cells. Most doctors recommend that this test be done twice a year after the age of thirty-five.

Breast Cancer. In the United States, breast cancer occurs more often and causes more deaths than any other kind of cancer. It is estimated that approximately ninety-five percent of breast cancers are discovered by the women themselves. This tells us why we should learn the technique of examining our own breasts for lumps. Only a physician can decide whether a lump requires a biopsy. If a biopsy is required, a portion of tissue is removed and examined under a microscope to determine whether the tumor is benign (noncancerous) or malignant (cancerous).

Waste no time in seeing your physician if you do find a lump. When the lump proves to be cancerous but is localized to the breast, it is estimated that about eighty-five percent of the treated patients have no signs of the disease at the end of five years. The following information gives the breast self-examination recommended by the American Cancer Society.

Breast self-examination should be done about one week after each menstrual period. Here are the steps:

1. Sit or stand in front of a mirror, your arms relaxed at your sides, and look for any changes in size, shape, and contour of the breasts. Also look for puckering or dimpling of the skin and changes on the surface of the nipples. Gently press each nipple to see if any discharge occurs.

2. Raise both arms over your head, and look for exactly the same things. Note differences since you last examined your breasts. (From here on you will be trying to find a lump or thickening.)

3. Lie down on your bed, put a pillow or a bath towel under your left shoulder, and your left hand under your head. With the fingers of your right hand held together and flat, press gently against the breast with small circular motions to feel the inner, upper portion of your left breast, starting at your breastbone and going outward toward the nipple line. Also feel the area around the nipple.

4. With the same gentle pressure, feel the lower inner part of your breast. Incidentally, in this area you may feel a ridge of firm tissue. Don't be alarmed. This is normal.

5. Now bring your left arm down to your side, and still using the flat part of the fingers of your right hand, feel under your left armpit.

6. Use the same gentle pressure to feel the upper, outer portion of your left breast from the nipple line to where your arm is resting.

7. Finally, feel the lower outer portion of your breast, going from the outer part to the nipple.

8. Repeat the entire procedure, as described, on the right breast using the left hand for the examination.

Cancer's Seven Warning Signals. The American Cancer Society has made it easy to learn cancer's seven warning signals. They begin with letters that spell the word "CAUTION" vertically:

*C*hange in bowel or bladder habits

A sore that does not heal

*U*nusual bleeding or discharge

*T*hickening or lump in breast or elsewhere

*I*ndigestion or difficulty in swallowing

*O*bvious change in wart or mole

*N*agging cough or hoarseness

Learn these warnings—they could save your life. If you have a warning signal that persists for two weeks, see your doctor.

FACTS ABOUT VENEREAL DISEASE

Sometimes even the most knowledgeable women do not know the facts about venereal disease, the social disease that is on the rampage in the United States today.

The following questions and answers are from material furnished by many state health departments for a venereal disease clinic's distribution.[2]

[2] "Fact Sheet on Venereal Disease," Houston City Health Department, Houston, Texas.

What Is VD? VD is the term used for venereal disease. The two most common forms of VD are syphilis and gonorrhea.

What Is Syphilis? Syphilis is a disease caused by an organism called a spirochete and can involve every part of the body.

How Is Syphilis Transmitted? Syphilis is transmitted at the time of sexual intercourse or intimate physical contact and may involve the sex organs, mouth, or rectum of an infected person.

What Are the Symptoms of Syphilis? In primary syphilis, the first sign of syphilis is a painless sore. It is most often found on or around the sex organs and usually appears from ten to ninety days (usually twenty-one days) after contact with an infected person.

Secondary Symptoms. The second signs of syphilis may appear between two to six months after contact. There may be a rash or skin eruption; persistent sore throat, fever, and headache; loss of patches of hair, or sores in the mouth.

The primary and secondary symptoms may disappear without medical treatment, but the disease is still present and will continue if left untreated.

Latent Syphilis. After the primary and secondary symptoms leave, the disease may become dormant for four to twenty-five years or longer if not treated. By this time the disease is strong within the body and may begin to attack the heart, brain, and spinal cord. A victim may become blind, insane, or crippled.

Can syphilis be cured? Syphilis can be cured with penicillin or other antibiotics. Even in the later stages of syphilis, one can be treated and cured of the disease. However, the damage already done to the body can never be repaired. Although the disease is curable, a person does not become immune, but can catch it again.

What Is Gonorrhea? Gonorrhea is the most common of the venereal diseases.[3] It is often called "the great sterilizer" because it attacks the reproductive system or rectum of the person.

How Is Gonorrhea Transmitted? Gonorrhea is usually transmitted at the time of sexual intercourse or intimate contact with the sex organs or rectum of an infected person.

---

[3]"Do You Know about the Most Commonly Reported Communicable Disease?" (New York: Pfizer Laboratories Division, Pfizer, Inc., May, 1971).

What Are the Symptoms of Gonorrhea? Males often experience painful urination accompanied by a discharge of pus. This occurs two to six days after contact with the infected person. A female rarely has symptoms. She may or may not have an increased vaginal discharge. Recent studies indicate that a small percentage of the males possibly do not have symptoms. Because of the lack of symptoms, the disease is spread unknowingly. In some population groups, one out of three may have this disease and not know it. A simple smear test confirms gonorrhea of the penis, but more complicated laboratory tests may be required in determining the presence of gonorrhea of the female sex organs or of the rectum.

Can Gonorrhea Be Cured? Gonorrhea is curable with antibiotics if it is treated early and under proper medical supervision. It is difficult to control and if not adequately treated it may progress to arthritis, sterility, heart problems, and painful pelvic disorders. Gonorrhea, like syphilis, can be caught often.

It is estimated that one hundred million people throughout the world have died of syphilis since 1900. More than $50,000,000 in tax monies are spent each year in the United States to support people who are insane or blind as a result of syphilis.

It is estimated that two million Americans were infected with venereal disease last year alone. This represents only part of the problem because many more cases go unreported.

Because the public has condemned the VD victim, the majority of states have passed laws allowing physicians to treat minors for these diseases without the knowledge or consent of their parents. These laws permit many minors to obtain medical care—many who would not otherwise because of parental reactions. But what about the innocent husband or wife whose promiscuous spouse has brought home a venereal disease? Even if a doctor is consulted, he often does not report the statistic because of his patient's humiliation.

In an effort to cut down the spread of venereal disease, some gynecologists routinely check their patients for it.

If you have questions regarding venereal disease, call your gynecologist or physician for an appointment, or stop by your city health department or venereal disease clinic. Your questions will be answered, and you will be given pamphlets upon request. Hopefully, knowledge of these facts may help prevent and cure venereal disease.

ENRICHMENT ACTIVITIES

1. Schedule for performing beauty routines: *Weekly*   *Daily*

    Hair: Shampoo and set   _____   _____

                 Pick-up curls   _____   _____

                 List the supplies needed: _____   _____

    Nails: Manicure   _____   _____

                 Pedicure   _____   _____

                 List the supplies needed: _____

    Beauty Bath: Do you prefer a shower or bath?

                                          _____   _____

                 Frequency: _____   _____

                 List bathing aids you consider essential: _____

                 List bathing aids you would like to have for added luxury: _____

2. Explain briefly how you select the "right" soap for your particular skin.

3. Why should cuticles on your toes and fingers be pushed back after each bath?

4. Which type of skin needs a moisturizer after a bath or shower?

5. Which type of fragrance is the strongest: cologne, toilet water, perfume, or sachet? Which type do you prefer? How do *you* select a perfume?

7. List fragrance "dos" you can remember

8. List fragrance "don'ts" you can remember.

9. Where are the apocrine glands located? Where are the eccrine glands located? Which gland produces a perspiration that can cause odor?

10. Explain the difference between a deodorant and an antiperspirant.

11. List the forms of deodorants.

12. How did you select your deodorant? How often do you apply it?

13. Do you use a feminine hygiene spray or powder? When do you use it and why is it important?

14. Do you wear sanitary napkins or tampons? How often do you change them?

15. List the methods of hair removal.

16. Do you have superfluous facial hair? By which method do you remove it?

17. How often do you remove the hair on your legs?

18. How often do you brush your teeth? When did you last see a dentist?

19. When did you last have a health checkup? List some of the things to be routinely checked by your doctor.

20. Have you ever had a Pap test? How often should you have a Pap test? Before age thirty-five? After age thirty-five?

21. List the seven warning signals of cancer. The word "caution" may help you.

C _____

A _____

U _____

T _____

I _____

O _____

N _____

22. Tell briefly how you should examine your breasts one week after your menstrual period.

23. Name the two most serious venereal diseases. How do you contract these diseases?

24. List the symptoms of syphilis. List the symptoms of gonorrhea.

25. Can syphilis be cured? Can you contract syphilis more than once?

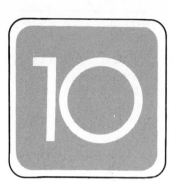

fashion sense

Every woman is involved in fashion. Fashion is many things: a means to cover your body, a tonic, an investment, a headache, a business, a hobby, an art. Is your fashion image good, bad, or indifferent? Thomas Fuller said, "Clothes don't make the man, but good clothes have gotten many a man a good job." The purpose of this chapter is to help you develop an individual fashion sense that will enhance you and your personality. Being well-dressed gives confidence, a quality that every woman needs. At the end of the chapter are some practical exercises that will help you in your fashion search.

Clothes may not make the woman, but they certainly tell the world about her. Many first and lasting impressions are created by how you present yourself in public—how you "put yourself together." Clothes make important impressions; they give clues about your personality, reveal your self-esteem, and reflect how you feel about others. What you wear should not only enhance your figure and suit the occasion, but should also harmonize with your personality. In Figure 73 the question is asked, "Do you know your personality type?" Are you a Sophisticated Extrovert, a Romantic Feminist, the Natural Athletic Type, or an Intellectual Individualist?

Your personality is affected by what you wear. Decide that you will look attractive at all times, and dress as carefully when you are staying at home as when you are going out to keep a business appointment. Don't think that you will not be seen when you dash to the grocery store. Your hair may be in rollers, and you may hope that no one will notice, so you tie a scarf around your head, and of course they won't see that dirty shirt (with a button missing) that you hope will cover the rip in your too tight pants. Because you're in a hurry, sloppy house shoes adorn your feet (besides, they feel good).

Everyone has shopping acquaintances: people encountered at the supermarket or shopping center, salespeople to whom you smile and say, "Hello." They may never know your name, but they know *you*. These people have been influenced by what you wear because this tells them about your personality. You may be saying, "But this isn't the real me." However, that is the only *you* they ever see. Remember, a moment can last forever.

The same principle is true regarding fellow workers. If you are spending several eight-to-ten-hour days, or the equivalent, at work, your dress is certain to be noticed, as it is in Figure 74. Your peers and executives make mental notes and verbal comments.

FIGURE 73.
Your image is showing.

FIGURE 74.
Personal grooming habits are as important as technical skills.

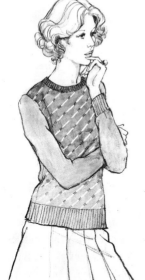

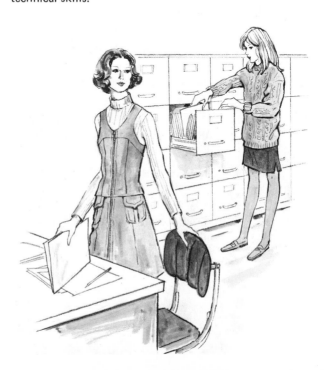

When our company was preparing for a seminar with an insurance company, the personnel director expressed concern about poor grooming habits of some of the women employees. He was very anxious about the company image; and distraught because some women were coming to work in houseshoes (big, fluffy ones, at that), no stockings, dresses that looked like housecoats, and with rollers in their hair. Of course, these women were in the minority, but remember, "It only takes one bad apple to spoil the barrel." A business is very protective of its image, and if you are an offender, you certainly can't complain if you never get out of the mailroom or never get a promotion when a vacancy occurs.

Most companies promote from among their employees when a position needs to be filled. Also, aggressive American businesses want to make, and are making, efforts to promote women to responsible positions.

In a large company, a man retired recently in the publications department and management decided to fill the position with one of the two women working in the department. Their records of performance were reviewed, and both women were found to be equally qualified. The decision was made on personal appearance. One woman was drab and unkempt in her appearance; the other was neat and attractively dressed. I'm sure you know who got the promotion: the woman who put herself together with thought and presented a good company image. Remember: In our national survey, businessmen agreed that personal grooming habits are equally as important as technical skills. A college dean when he was recently speaking about some classes, made this statement: "Everyone is hired because of his skills. Whether or not he keeps that job depends on the presence or failure of attitudes and grooming habits. And if he is a two-time offender, he won't have the third opportunity."

There is an age-old question, "Should a woman dress to please men, women, or herself?" Possibly you think the previous statements advocate dressing for others. Not really. Dress to please yourself as much as you dress to please others, but even better than that, dress to enhance yourself as an individual. There is quite a difference between pleasing and enhancing, and with the difference comes responsibility. Acquire good judgment, and know when to wear jeans, shorts, and décolleté dresses. A secretary stated recently that if she has a hangover and feels perfectly miserable, she goes to the office in jeans and tennis shoes. You can admire her boss' sense of humor, but not his fashion sense. The rewards of dressing to benefit yourself as an individual will be a more handsome you, recognition, and confidence.

You may have asked the question, "How do I know the fashions that are right for me?" There are some very basic facts you must know about yourself: your figure type and what colors look best on you, always keeping in mind your lifestyle. Have an adventuresome spirit and be interested in yourself.

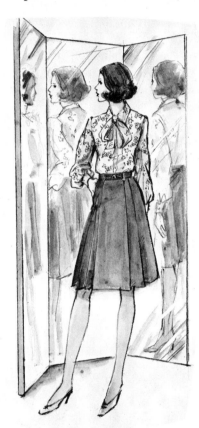

FIGURE 75.
It is imperative that you look just as good going as you do coming.

A full-length mirror is important. If you don't have one, invest in one immediately and look at yourself before going out. And don't forget to look at the back view as shown in Figure 75. Have you ever stopped to think how many people walk behind you every day? There may be hundreds who seldom, if ever, see you from the front. It is imperative that you look as good going as you do coming.

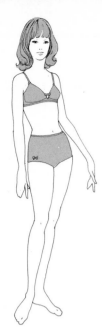

FIGURE 76.

KNOW YOUR FIGURE TYPE

It is safe to say there are no two figures exactly alike. Mother Nature has given women an endless combination of shoulders, busts, waists, hips, legs, and bone structures, making each one of us unique. Rare is the woman who is born with a perfect body line. For decades American women have tried to remain slim but not curveless. This "ideal American look" has motivated many women to join exercise and diet clubs. In a well-proportioned figure, shown in Figure 76, the bust and hip measurements are exactly the same with the waist ten inches smaller, and the total bulk of the body is in correct proportion to the total height. The shoulders should not be too wide or too narrow, the waist neither too low nor too high.

At this point it might be wise to reflect on how men feel about women's figures. First of all, it goes without saying: They like figures! In surveys taken among men, almost all of them admit they do not want their woman to have a fashion model figure. They like women who look real and believable, who have shape and roundness. The next time you wish for the figure you see in a magazine, remember that the camera adds ten pounds. On the other hand, if you are pudgy and overweight, don't kid yourself into believing he likes you for what you are and not how you look. Another myth is that fat people are happy people. In Chapter Eight you learned what diet and exercise will do for your figure. And remember, no matter what your figure type and problems are, good posture is also essential.

Most figure types fall into the following three catagories:

Tall: 5'9" and over, with thin, medium, or heavy body frame
Moderate: 5'4" through 5'8", with thin, medium, or heavy body frame
Short: under 5'3", with thin, medium, or heavy body frame

Take a good, honest look at yourself in that full-length mirror. Look at yourself from the front, sides, and back without your clothes on (it could be a shock). Then, in your foundation garments, bathing suit, or leotards, take your bust, waist, and hip measurements. Become aware of your figure problems and find ways to camouflage them. Please don't take the defeatist attitude and declare that there is nothing that can be done. Every problem has a solution. The solutions can be found in the line, color, and fabric of your clothes, foundation garments, and mental attitude.

THE EFFECT OF LINE

In Chapter Seven "Poise in Motion," you learned that to have good carriage you must stand tall, sit tall, walk tall, and think tall. To achieve total figure flattery you should dress tall, as well.

In seminars conducted by CPI, thousands of women have indicated their desire to be taller, and almost as many have expressed a wish to be shorter. This wish could often be granted if they would carefully study the clothes they wear. In order to create the desired illusion of height, you need to master the art of figure camouflage.

In discussing wardrobe, *line* refers to the shape and cut of a garment. By capitalizing upon line and using it to your best advantage, you emphasize your good features and minimize your poor ones. In clothing, a line can be created by seams in a dress or jacket, pockets, buttons, braid, rows of tucking, a deep hem, contrasting colors of bands, belts, yokes, pleats, gathers, fabric patterns, necklaces, scarves, or the angle of a hat. Lines can be straight or curved. Refer to Figure 77.

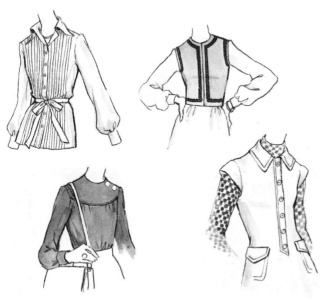

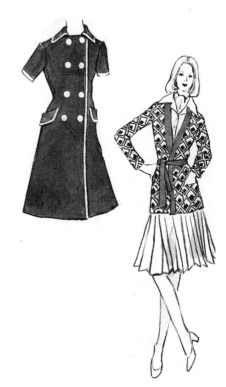

FIGURE 77.
Lines in clothing are created by details.

The eye will follow a line; therefore several lines together can cause an optical illusion. You can create an optical illusion by having lines going in different directions on your figure.

The lines in Figure 78 are the same length. They appear to be different because of the added short lines. On the opposite set, the same short lines are drawn at the bottom. Now the lines appear even shorter or longer. Draw a dress silhouette several times and add lines at different places and angles. Notice that the dress looks longer, shorter, or wider.

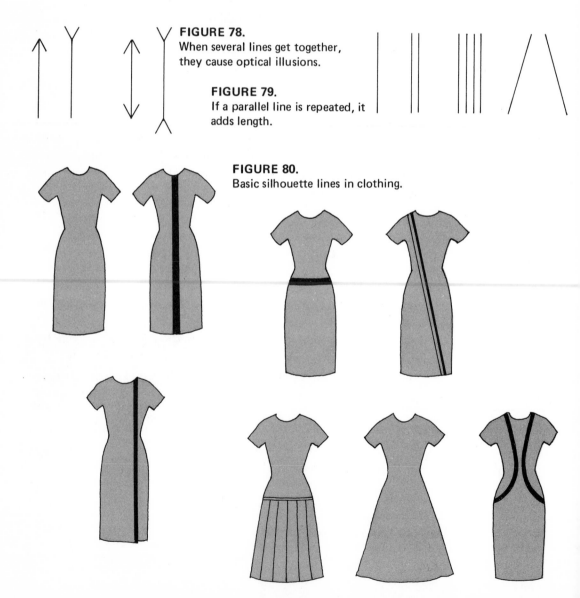

FIGURE 78.
When several lines get together, they cause optical illusions.

FIGURE 79.
If a parallel line is repeated, it adds length.

FIGURE 80.
Basic silhouette lines in clothing.

If parallel lines are repeated, it adds width, as illustrated in Figure 79. If same-length lines angle toward one another, they appear even wider and shorter in height. See Figure 80 for the basic silhouette lines.

There are many different figure types—we have already named nine—and for each there is a special way to dress. Here are a few guidelines for tall and short women. However, if you are heavy, not all of these principles will apply to you. If you are 5'9" or over and thin or medium, you can take any liberties with your clothes. You certainly don't have to cut your height to look shorter if you don't want to. On the other hand, if you are under 5'3", you will want to acquire an illusion of height.

Short (5'3" and Under):

1. Wear clothes and accessories in proportion to your petite size. Remember you are striving to appear taller.
2. Wear clothes with simple, dainty trimmings. Too much gathering or trim will weigh you down.
3. Keep your silhouette slim and smooth. The princess and empire lines are good for you.
4. Wear soft, smooth fabrics. Avoid heavy fabrics, organdy, and other stiff materials.
5. Suits should have short jackets or boleros. Avoid long jackets and tunics.
6. Jackets and skirts should be the same color. A jacket of one color and a skirt of another will cut your figure in half.
7. Select clothes with vertical lines that are not broken by trim and belts.
8. Belts should be narrow and of the same fabric as your dress. Avoid wide, contrasting ones with large buckles and heavy trim.
9. Wear small prints rather than large prints and bold plaids.
10. Coats should be full-length, fitted, or boxy. Avoid big pockets and large collars.
11. Skirts should be straight or gently flared. Too much fullness will overpower you.
12. Accessories should be small or medium-sized. Avoid large handbags of contrasting color and a lot of clutter.

13. Wear shoes with medium-high heels. Avoid heels that are too high or very flat.

Tall (5'9" and Over):

1. Choose clothes with horizontal lines.
2. Select accessories of contrasting colors and unusual designs, also large purses, and heavy jewelry.
3. Wear jackets and skirts of contrasting colors and materials to break the line. Double-breasted jackets are especially good.
4. Wide belts of contrasting colors are better than narrow belts.
5. Wear skirts that are gored, pleated, or gathered. Avoid skimpy ones.
6. Wear clothes of good proportion, and avoid skimpiness and bagginess. Good fit is extremely important.
7. Select figured materials rather than fabrics of a solid color.
8. Bold prints and plaids are good.
9. Wear a fitted or belted coat. Wide lapels, big pockets, large collars, and deep cuffs are all good.
10. Strive for sophistication in your dress.
11. Choose shoes with medium heels.

In the study of makeup, you learned the techniques for creating the illusion of an oval face if yours is not oval naturally. When selecting jewelry and the neckline of a dress, you can also soften your face shape, or create the illusion of a longer or shorter neck by following a few simple guidelines. Because repetition emphasizes, do not repeat a line—in the neckline of a dress or in jewelry—that you do not wish to emphasize in your face. We do not advocate that an oval face is the most perfect facial shape. Many classically beautiful women have rectangular, square, and heart-shaped faces. Actually, this can be a dramatic feature. If your face is anything but oval, don't feel that nature dealt you a bad card. Capitalize on your dramatic features. But there will always be women who want to minimize the face shape for various reasons; and the following points, some of which are illustrated in Figure 81, should be considered when you are selecting jewelry and necklines.

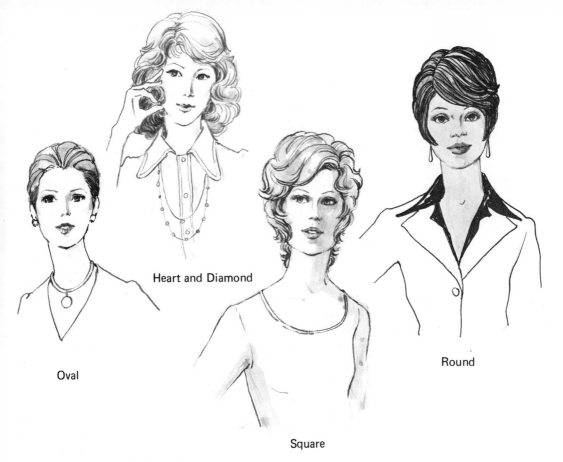

Heart and Diamond

Oval

Square

Round

FIGURE 81.
Select necklines and jewelry to flatter your face shape.

Oval face:	Wear the necklines and jewelry you desire.
Square face:	Wear round or V-necklines. If you have a dress with a square neckline, soften it with a scarf or necklace. A collar or pin in the center will make the face seem more oval. Avoid square earrings; drop earrings create a vertical line if your face is very wide.
Round face:	Choose square and V-necklines, pointed collars, and narrow lapels. Avoid turtlenecks, oval necklines, and round collars. In jewelry, avoid round, ball earrings; round pins; and tight choker necklaces.
Rectangular face:	Wear high, round necklines. You can wear ruffles, turtleneck and mandarin collars, bateau necklines, chokers, scarves, ascots, cluster and ball earrings. Avoid square, V, and U-shaped necklines;

175

square earrings and pins; and pendants on long chains.

Heart-Shaped or Diamond-Shaped face: These two face types can wear the same jewelry and necklines. Wear high, round, and oval necklines. Added ruffles and rolled collars add balance. Avoid the deep V-neckline and long necklaces.

THE EFFECT OF COLOR

What artist hasn't been inspired by the colors of the rainbow bouncing off a green mountain, gleaming in the bright sunlight, and fading into the blue sky; or looking at a green meadow filled with patches of bright, cool wild flowers? Countless women have been tantalized when shopping or thumbing through fashion magazines by the endless combinations of colors available for their wardrobes.

All the colors in the world can now be yours, thanks to twentieth-century technology. Manufacturers can produce any imagined color on various fabrics at a price you can afford. Color is no longer restricted to a season; white and pastels are worn twelve months a year, and black and chocolate brown will compliment any summer tan. Color combinations are only restricted by your

FIGURE 82.
The color wheel. Develop a good eye for color and see it for what it is.

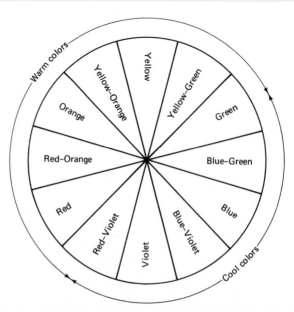

imagination. Do you remember how alive you felt the first time you saw pink and orange together and then again with purple?

Every well-planned wardrobe must have a basic color as its foundation. Basic colors are no longer just black, brown, and blue. These are still great colors to use, but today you have other choices such as gray, camel, and even red. This is possible because of the new freedom you have in color coordination.

In choosing your colors you will be restricted only by these factors: color of your hair and eyes, skin tone, figure type, and your basic wardrobe color.

The Color Wheel. The colors of the color wheel were first arranged by Sir Isaac Newton. The primary colors are red, yellow, and blue. The secondary colors are green, orange, and violet, made by mixing equal amounts of two of the primary colors. No combination of colors can produce red, yellow, or blue. The color harmonies are a combination of a primary color and the neighboring secondary color. They are yellow-green, blue-green, blue-violet, red-violet, red-orange, and yellow-orange. Figure 82 shows the relationship of the colors on the color wheel.

Study the twelve bright colors on a color wheel and become familiar with the endless variations of the tints and shades. Develop a good eye for color, and see it for what it is. Red will no longer be just red; it will be rose, pink, scarlet, burgundy, or maroon. If it has been a long time since you've played with watercolors, it will be good for you to perform this experiment. Paint a pure color, such as blue, in the center of a piece of paper. Gradually add white to the blue, and paint successively lighter tints until it becomes the palest of blues. Add black little by little, painting after each addition to the pure color, and paint it on the other side of the blue in the center of the page until it becomes charcoal. You should have about ten different shades and tints on your paper. In fashion coordinating this is called monotoning: using a succession of tints and shades of a base color. Use this new sense of color to coordinate a new outfit the next time you add to your wardrobe.

Color and Your Skin. When you studied makeup, you analyzed your coloring and learned your skin tone. For review, the colorings are: cool skin with blue undertones; warm skin with yellow undertones; natural skin that has pink and beige undertones; and dark complexions with brown, red-brown, and golden tones.

Your skin and facial coloring are the most important factors in selecting your best color. You need a color that will make your skin look healthy and clear. The color needs to be lighter or darker than the value of your skin tone. This applies to all skin, no matter what its balance. The undertones of your skin should be the same as the underlying tones of the color you wear. For example, a blonde with cool skin will look especially pleasing in pale blues, reds, and greens that have blue in them. A warm-skinned brunette will look her best in shades that have a yellow tint; a natural skin with pink undertones usually look best in shades that have a tint of red or blue in them. Dark complexions look very good in strong colors, especially yellows, reds, and grayed-down shades of deep colors.

Important tips to remember:

1. Black, gray, and brown will drain color from your face.
2. Pastel and grayed-down shades flatter pale skins.
3. Intense shades drain color from your face.
4. Do not wear an unbecoming color next to your face.
5. Blue, violet, and gray create shadows. Avoid these if your skin has blemishes, wrinkles, or dark circles under your eyes.
6. The colors you wear should be in perfect harmony with your makeup and nail polish.
7. If you change the color of your hair or makeup, it will affect the colors of fabric you should wear.

Color and Your Eyes. Your eyes are emphasized when you wear a color that match them or that is slightly darker. They will reflect the color you wear. Brown eyes are emphasized by brown and orange tones, blue eyes by blue, and green eyes by green. If your eyes are hazel, containing several colors, highlight the strongest color.

Color and Your Hair. To flatter your hair, choose colors that enhance rather than detract from the hair color. Complementary colors, those that fall opposite each other on a color wheel, will intensify your hair color. When selecting a harmonizing shade, be careful that it is not too vivid a hue, which might steal the attention.

Color and Your Figure. Use color in your wardrobe to emphasize the good points of your figure and to minimize your figure faults. Remember: Light colors reflect light and dark colors absorb light. This is why you look larger in a light colored dress and smaller in a dark dress. If your hips are too large don't wear a white skirt, which will emphasize them. On the other hand, if your hips are small and you want them to appear larger, do wear a white or light colored skirt. Figure 83 shows how the use of two colors in the right places in a costume will help to conceal a figure fault. If you are top-heavy, wear a dark color in the bodice of your costume and a light color in the skirt. If you have too much weight in the hip area and are bottom-heavy, reverse the order: light colors above the waist and dark below. The use of two colors can make a figure appear shorter and wider. One-color costumes can add height.

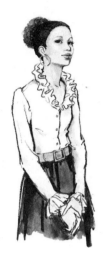
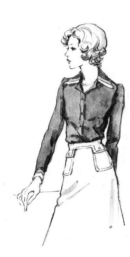

FIGURE 83.
Use color to flatter your figure. Because of light reflection, you look larger in light colors and smaller in dark colors.

Color and Psychological Impact. If you have been relying on the clasic "little black dress" and gray flannel suit to carry you through a season, you have been using good taste. However, no woman should stay in the black, brown, and gray syndrome all her life. You owe it to yourself and your audience to study the exciting world of color and learn how to make it work to your advantage. Keep the following facts in mind:

1. Color attacts attention.
2. Color creates an illusion of height and size.
3. Color creates moods.
4. Color can complement your personality.

Psychologists say that the colors you like and dislike tell a lot about your personality. If you are an extrovert and are sought as a leader, you usually prefer the vivid, dominant colors. A person who selects soft and pastel colors is considered demure and soothing.

Colors are classified as warm or cool in their psychological effect. Reds and yellows, warm colors, are stimulating; and cool colors, greens and blues, are calming.

BECOME A FASHION PERCEIVER

A flair for fashions cannot be bought, but it can be acquired by paying close attention to the wealth of material and experiences that are available to you. How many times have you sat down to relax and thumb through a fashion magazine for enjoyment, then closed it and put it aside and that was that? To perceive what is going on in the fashion world and how you can use it to your best advantage, pay close attention to trends and details and analyze what designers are saying. Your best sources for this information are fashion

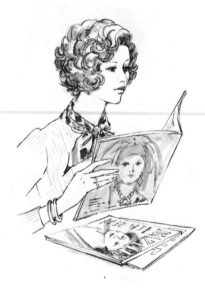

FIGURE 84.
Adapt available fashion information to your needs.

magazines, newspaper ads of the better stores and shops, window displays of fashionable stores, a friend or celebrity whose fashion flair you admire, designer styleshows, and "The Best of the Season" styleshows coordinated in many department stores (which, by the way, are free). Naturally you will not be able to buy everything you see and like, but with a discerning eye you will understand how what you see can work for you, the individual. Things to look for would be the length and shape of skirts, length and shape of jackets and sleeves, necklines, new fashion colors, combinations of colors, fabrics, and accessories, lines in coats and jackets, and for what occasion to wear the clothes.

Have fun in your new fashion study. Make mental and written notes, even dogear the pages in your magazines, and begin to analyze what is right for you. Refer to Figure 84.

1. Determine the amount of money you will spend on your season's wardrobe.

2. Is the "new fashion color" good on you? If not, forget about it. Consider spending small amounts on a scarf or jewelry.

3. Are the current fashion lines good for your figure? If not, stay with your tried and proven lines.

4. Are the accessories (shoes, stockings, handbags, belts, scarves, hats, and jewelry) flattering to you? If they are too big and would overpower you, shop for them in a smaller size.

5. Do the current fashions blend with your personality, life style, and geographical location?

"A Fashion Perceiver is one who avails herself of all available fashion information and then is able to adapt this information to her individual needs, using personal appearance, personal activities, monetary status, and geographical location as her tools for adaptation."[1] When you have learned and applied these principles, you will be decorously dressed. Good taste is a sense of rightness—a refined look. It is a conservative rather than a dramatic look; it is simplicity. Remember: You wear the clothes; the clothes do not wear you.

Fashion or Fad. Learn to discern between fashion and fad. Fad is fun, but it is also expensive if you shop on a budget. Fad is a fashion that lasts one season and then becomes outdated, for example, knickers, hot pants, and the midi. You can probably name others that are hanging in your closet. Good fashion has simple, classic lines, and can be worn for several years without looking dated.

[1] Jean Adams, "Total Woman," United Features Syndicate.

It is an outfit that can take several accessory changes to suit particular occasions, therefore stretching your fashion dollar.

INVENTORY YOUR WARDROBE

The classic statement that every woman has made at one time or another is, "I don't have anything to wear," even though she may have a closet or chest full of clothes as in Figure 85. Spend a profitable day by taking an inventory of your clothes and accessories. Organize your wardrobe into categories: work, play, and evening. Put each dress, suit, skirt, blouse, and coat into its proper category. Lay out your accessories: shoes, handbags, belts, stockings, scarves, and jewelry. You may find you have a red skirt and no blouse to wear with it or a navy dress and no shoes to complement it. In order to get a good picture of what you have and what you need to give your wardrobe the finishing touches, fill in a chart like Chart 3. You may be surprised at how many blanks you leave. But now you will know where you need to add to your wardrobe to spend your fashion dollar wisely.

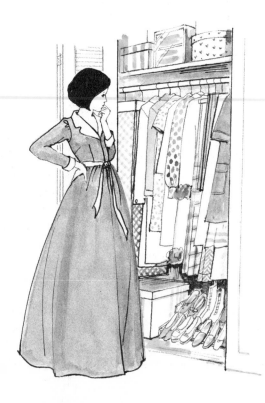

FIGURE 85.
Take an inventory of your clothes and accessories, and organize your closet.

CHART 3

Your Wardrobe Inventory Chart

Suits, Dresses, Separates, Pant Suits	Shoes	Handbags	Accessories	Foundation Garments
1.				
2.				
3.				
4.				
5.				
6.				
7.				
8.				
9.				
10.				
11.				
12.				

BE A WISE SHOPPER

Do you like everything you wear? If you can answer affirmatively, we want to be the first to congratulate you because of the individual fashion flair you have developed. However, most women make unwise purchases and have "dogs" hanging in their closets. On the other hand, you probably have some favorite outfits you enjoy wearing; you feel good in them and receive compliments from your associates on how terrific you look. Analyze the reasons for the success of these outfits. What is the color? What is the line of the dress, shape of the neckline, shape of the skirt, placement of the waist, length of the jacket, shape of the sleeve? How do you use accessories with them? All of these factors add up to why the costume is right for you. Now you have a working idea of what colors, lines, and accessories enhance your figure.

Shopping is a very important key to fashion success. Figure 86 shows a wise shopper. Whether you realize it or not, you are a vital part of one of the biggest businesses in the United States. Every year mammoth cash registers ring up billions of dollars paid to the dress industry alone. Think about the sales in all the related industries! Fashion is an investment. Are you investing wisely? The following are some points to consider when you shop.

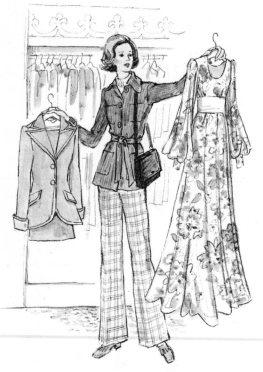

FIGURE 86.
Make wise decisions and purchases when you shop.

1. *Don't buy any old time the spirit moves.* There are some women who, when they have "the blues," go out to buy something. They consider a hat or dress a great picker-upper, only to find later that it doesn't go with a thing in the wardrobe; another day they may even wonder why they made the purchase.

2. *Don't shop in a hurry.* We all know "haste makes waste." Many busy people must take advantage of shopping on their lunch hour or in a few minutes squeezed into the day. If this is how you do most of your purchasing, plan ahead. Make a list of your needs, and get ideas from fashion magazines and newspapers of what is available

before you go shopping. Try looking one day and, after thinking about what you have seen, go back to buy.

3. *Know your figure type.* By now you should know what dress lines are most suitable for you. This will save time. As you look through the racks, you will have an idea of which dress to try on and which to avoid.

4. *Wear new fashions only if they are becoming to you.*

5. *Don't buy clothes or accessories just because they are on sale.* If you can take advantage of a sale and save money, certainly that is advisable. But if you buy a dress at one-fifth of the original price and you don't have shoes or bag to match, how wise is your purchase? Have you really saved money?

6. *Wear proper foundation garments when shopping.* How many times have you tried on a skirt and said to yourself, "When I have my girdle on, it will look better." Don't rely on the clothes' looking better when you look better. Also remember to wear stockings, shoes in good repair, well-applied makeup, and have your hair neat and clean. A well-dressed woman will attract the attention of a saleslady, and the saleslady will be more anxious to help you.

7. *Don't buy a complete outfit in one day.* Total coordination of an outfit takes thought and time. It is wise to select the costume, dress, suit, or separates first, and then select the accessories. There are several factors involved in coordinating an outfit: planning, time, and budget. It is wise to purchase the costume and select the accessories later. Unwise choices can be made at the end of a day when time is short and you are tired.

8. *Don't buy shoes in the afternoon.* Rarely do shoes feel good on tired, aching feet. Buy your shoes when your body is fresh and you can determine if the shoes are a good fit. Then, if the shoes hurt, you will know it is the shoes and not your feet.

9. *Select clothes that fit your lifestyle.* If you are a career woman, the major portion of your fashion dollar should be spent on clothes you can wear to the office, and the balance on casual wear and clothes for evenings in or out. Don't overload your wardrobe with frilly chiffons and

pants that will do you no good at eight a.m. when you are dressing for work, or the time will come when you look into your closet and exclaim, "I never have anything to wear."

10. *Buy well-constructed clothes.* Develop a discerning eye for quality workmanship. Check the seams to see if they are straight and sewn with close stitches. The seam allowance inside the garment should be at least five-eighths of an inch. Look at the buttonholes and make sure that one pull on a loose thread won't fray the edges. Bound buttonholes always give a finished look. Are the buttons, belt, and zipper of good quality? The hem should be at least two or three inches deep, depending on the fabric and skirt shape. The fabric should have a hard or sturdy finish and be wrinkle-free and soil resistant. A slim skirt constructed of loosely woven fabric should be lined.

11. *Remember your budget.* It has been said that American women can have designer clothes at one-tenth the original price. You can find well-constructed clothes with good design without spending a lot of money. The most expensive items in your wardrobe will be your coat, suit, and multiple-piece ensemble. If you have a weakness for shoes, handbags, or lingerie, be careful not to spend too much in this area. Remember to include in your budget the expense of clothing upkeep: cleaning, repairs, and replacement.

YOUR BASIC WARDROBE

You have learned the fundamentals of line, color, and shopping, and now you are ready to build your basic wardrobe, coordinated clothes that will carry you through all seasons and to all occasions with ease and confidence. These basic clothes will make it possible for you to always have something appropriate to wear, whether you are going to work or to a formal dinner.

Once again, remember that you wear the clothes; the clothes do not wear you. Good taste in clothes selection can be defined as elegant simplicity. The fewer frills and buttons you have on a costume, the more freedom you have in accessorizing. Fashion-wise clothes do not tell the world what season they appeared on the designer's board or what year you bought them. You will be able to wear a well-selected suit or dress from three to five years without its looking dated. The key word is *plan*.

Start by filling in the Personal Analysis Chart (Chart 4) to guide you in planning your basic wardrobe.

CHART 4

Personal Analysis Chart

Height _____

Weight _____

Measurements _____

Size of your body frame _____

Shape of your face _____

Length of your neck _____

Color of your eyes _____

Color of your hair _____

Skin tone _____

Fabrics you wear well _____

Your best color _____

Your best lines _____

Life style _____

Begin your planning by deciding which one of the basic colors will determine your color scheme. At times, the neutral colors—beige, gray, or tan—can serve as alternates. If you select brown as your basic color, this does not mean everything must be brown, beige, or white; but they must be colors that are flattering to you and that can be worn with brown.

Plan your wardrobe around your most expensive item: coat, suit, or costume. This item should be simple in line and style and in a solid color, either your basic color or a netural that will blend with every color in your wardrobe. If chosen wisely, it will be suitable to wear for the broadest range of activities in your professional and personal worlds. When selecting a suit, think of how adaptable it will be to blouses; choose tailored blouses for business and silks or chiffons for evening.

Today your fashion dollar will be spent wisely on a multiple-piece garment. This costume could be a combination of three or four of the following: skirt, pants, blouse, dress, jacket, vest, sleeveless jacket, and even a belt or scarf. Not all the pieces need be a solid color; one or two might be a coordinated stripe or plaid. If you choose your purchases wisely, you can plan your season's wardrobe around them with excitement and versatility. You should never have to feel you are putting on the "same old thing" again.

Your basic dress should be in one of the basic colors. The dress should be a classic silhouette in design and constructed of a wrinkle-free fabric. Its neckline should be neither too low nor too high, and should take to scarves, jewelry, or collars. It should have sleeves, and the buttons and belt should be self-covered.

Select basic shoes, handbag, and gloves of good leather and in one of the basic colors. If blue is your basic color, your shoes and handbag must be blue. Shoes should be free of buckles and contrasting stitching. A variety of buckles can be purchased to add to your shoes for a change.

Every wardrobe needs separates—blouses, sweaters, skirts, and jackets—for variety. Just a few well-chosen pieces can give the spark of versatility you need. Plan them to coordinate with your dresses and suits. This might be called "fashion on a budget," as illustrated in Figure 87.

A career woman's basic wardrobe should include the following:

Coat and accessories in a basic color
Shoes and purse of good leather
Good suit or multiple-piece ensemble
Basic dress
Basic dressy dress
Jumper
Basic pant suit
Blouses and skirts to mix and match

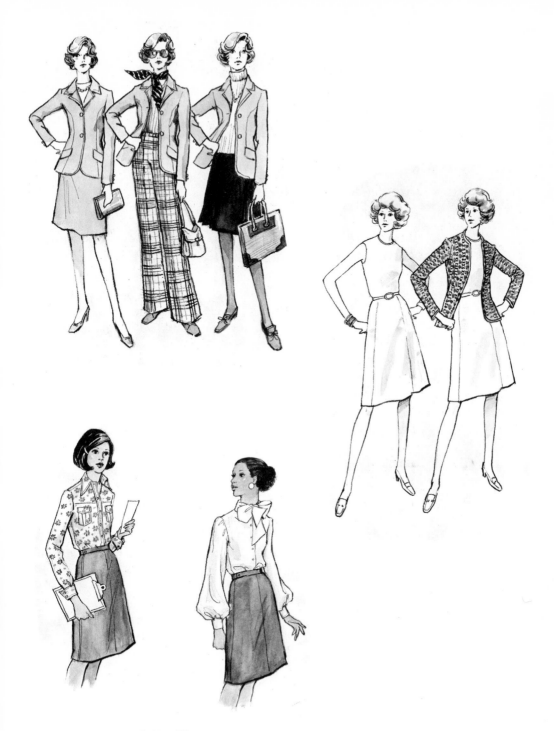

FIGURE 87.
There is a minimum of twelve outfits that can be coordinated from these few basic pieces. Find them.

Change of shoes
Gloves to coordinate with your basic color
One or two sweaters
A few less expensive dresses or pant suits
A few scarves
One or two belts
Jewelry—gold, silver, and pearls
Hats

ACCESSORIES ARE THE KEY

There is no question about it: Accessories can make or break the total effect of an ensemble. Your accessories reveal your personality and your cleverness with color and fashions. In a basic, limited wardrobe, smart accessories are a wise investment. They should be versatile enough to be worn with several outfits. You would be wise to become an accessory collector. Watch for sales, or when you have some extra money, invest in a handsome leather bag or a smart piece of jewelry that looks like the "real thing," or maybe a real-fur turban.

These are the basic rules of color combinations used to achieve a handsome look.

1. Monochromatic color tones—everything in the ensemble will be a tint or shade of one basic color.
2. Wear one color predominately with one single use of a second color.
3. Wear two colors on the body and a different base for the accessories.

Remember that white and black are considered neutrals and may be worn as a third color. Three colors should be the limit, and there will be times when two are best. The exception is when you wear a print or plaid of many colors. Following are a few simple rules that even the fashion experts follow.

1. Keep accessories and dress in the same category. The total effect should be one of harmony.
2. With dramatic clothes, use simple and very few accessories.

3. Understated clothes of solid colors can take dramatic jewelry and some patterned accessories.
4. A print costume needs solid-colored accessories.
5. Generally, the darkest color in the dress determines the color of the shoe.
6. Accent dark colors with light colors and vice versa.
7. Bright, vivid colors are best accented with neutrals.

Figure 88 shows the seven accessory points to consider when coordinating an ensemble. But please, don't try to hang something on all seven places just because they are available.

Head: Select hats that flatter your face shape and colors that are a good contrast to your coloring. Scarves can be worn as turbans or tied in a band around your hair. Earrings can be the perfect touch, but remember your face shape.

Neck: Depending on the neckline of your dress, a pin, necklace, rope, pendant, or scarf is a good addition to an outfit.

Waist: Belts come in all sizes, shapes, and colors, and if your figure can carry one, wear it with pride. A scarf can be worn at the waist.

Arms: Bracelets and watches should be worn in good taste to enhance the mood of your outfit.

Hand: Your selection of handbag will either enhance or detract from your total image. Remember your figure type when selecting the size and color. Gloves are important for the finished look. The length of the glove depends on the length of the dress sleeve.

Legs: Don't be guilty of buying one shade of hose to wear year round with everything in your wardrobe. The shade of your hose should be color-keyed to your costume. Even support hose come in fashion colors, and many well-dressed women wear them. If you are on your feet a lot, try them. Also wear them under your slacks for control. Many women have replaced their girdles with support hose.

Feet: Never before have shoes been more exciting. You have every shape and color from which to choose. For you to be well-dressed, your shoes must be color-coordinated and in good repair.

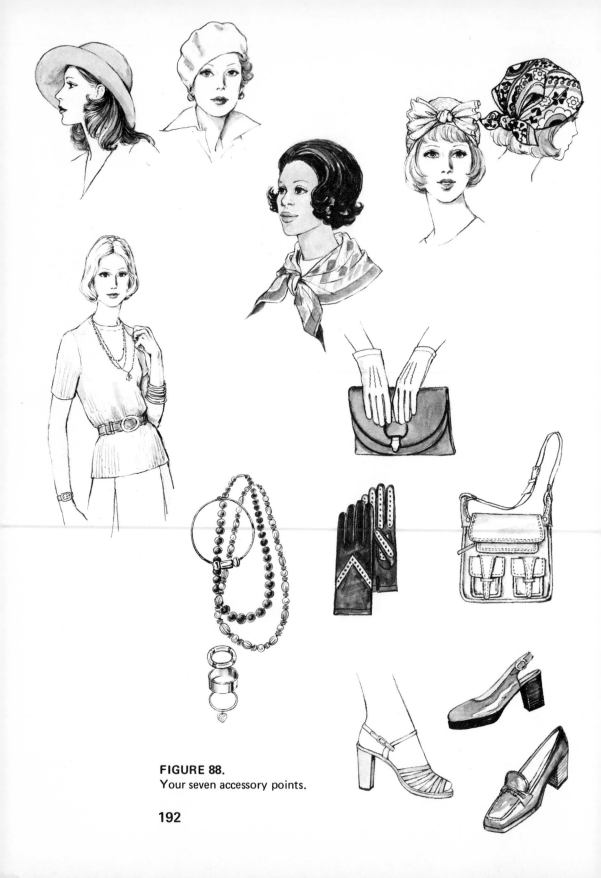

FIGURE 88.
Your seven accessory points.

192

It would be an impossible task to tell you what accessories are best for you. A line from a Broadway musical asks, "Does anyone still wear hats?" You may have the same feeling about gloves, too. The new freedom in fashions has certainly eliminated the necessity of wearing white gloves and prim hats. However, in some geographical locations hats and gloves are a must. And there is a cycle in fashions; many influences that are gone today will return tomorrow. Choosing accessories is an individual matter, and it is up to you to determine what items and colors will add the finishing touches and versatility to your costume. You will need to try different ideas, and with experience you will achieve that total look of elegant simplicity.

ENRICHMENT ACTIVITIES

1. Perform the activities suggested in the chapter and fill in the charts.
2. List ways of selecting clothes to camouflage your particular figure faults. Find examples from magazines or pattern books, and paste them into a notebook. (Pattern books can be purchased from fabric shops for a nominal fee.)
3. Obtain a color wheel, and learn how color works.
4. Experiment with creating color schemes, using water colors, acrylic paints, or color slides.
5. Make your personal color analysis and determine which colors you can wear.
6. Plan a basic wardrobe for summer and for winter.
7. Plan three outfits—casual, dress, and after-five—using your best colors. Either paint them in a notebook or find examples in magazines, and paste cutouts into your notebook.
8. Find the eight basic silhouette dress lines and paste them into the notebook.
9. Find examples of one or more of the silhouette lines combined in a single dress.
10. Attend at least two fashion shows, one of a designer's collection. Write your impressions of what the designers have created.

11. Determine the fashion fad of the day.
12. What are your best sizes in dresses, skirts, blouses, sweaters, pants, coats, gloves, and shoes?

three

business
image

professional
behavior

When you have graduated from your chosen educational program, the ideal is to know the kind of work you want to do in life. It makes good sense to do the type of work that you do well, work that you enjoy doing, and for which you have been trained. Life is too precious to fill with doing work that might make you, as well as those around you, miserable. Aptitude tests will be helpful if you are having difficulty determining which path to follow. Check with your local college, high school counselor, or state employment commission for types and costs of these aptitude tests. In many cases, they are free.

ARRANGING THE JOB INTERVIEW

Once you have decided what kind of job you want, it is time to get busy setting up interviews. There are several ways to go about arranging an interview.

Personal Contacts. Let people know the kind of job you are seeking. Friends or acquaintances can be extremely helpful in putting you onto possible job leads or by giving you an entree into a company or firm. Most people are very happy to help friends find jobs. Don't be too hurt, however, if some are not so anxious to help. Some people are hesitant to recommend a person for a job for fear that if it doesn't work out well, they may be blamed.

197

Don't be too smug about the personal and inside "contacts" who *do* help. Never misuse these contacts. They should simply be a steppingstone toward the job. If the company or firm is the type of well-run business that you would want to be a part of, the capable interviewer will consider you and your qualifications and discount the contact. You will have to sell the interviewer on yourself and your qualifications. This is particularly true if it is a "courtesy" interview for a "friend of a friend." Don't try to impress the interviewer with *who* you know, but with *what* you know.

Newspaper Ads. You may follow up employment ads in your newspaper. If the job is well-defined and seems to be the type of position you are seeking, waste no time in finding out more about it. Call if there is a number, or send a letter and résumé inquiring about the position. There is an advantage to newspaper ads because you know there is a definite job opening or the ad would not have been placed.

Employment Agencies. Be sure to choose a reputable agency that has broad coverage of job listings and firms. This will facilitate your placement into a position compatible with your experience, education, and job desires. Most reputable employment agencies have well-trained interviewers who will work diligently to please you as well as the firms they represent. However, some agencies have so few listings that they will try to place you in any available opening they have listed, whether it suits you or not. Employment agencies usually require a percentage of your first month's or first year's income. However, many companies now pay this fee for their new employees. State employment commissions can also be very helpful in locating jobs. There is no fee charged for their services.

If one of the above three methods does not produce a job, make a list of all the business concerns in your city that may be involved in the type of work you want. You can gather this list from the yellow pages of the telephone directory, or from the business directory in your local library.

Next, call these businesses and get the proper name and correct spelling of the personnel director or interviewer. Send a letter and a résumé to each one, telling him the type of job you are seeking as well as the qualifications you have to offer the company. In a few days, follow up on the telephone and ask if an interview can be arranged. Do not be a pest, but remember that persistence has landed many a job.

THE RÉSUMÉ

A résumé is a biographical sketch of personal data, your educational background, and your business experience. If you have had very little or no business experience it would be wise to confine the résumé to one page. Personnel directors are more likely to read a one-page résumé than a longer one.

In most instances, the interviewer sees the résumé before he sees you. Therefore, you want it to accomplish on paper what you later hope to confirm in person during an interview. It should be written for the particular job you are seeking, placing emphasis on your qualifications that would be compatible with and helpful in that position.

The résumé should be typed and readable with spaces between sections or categories of information. An original typed résumé should be neat and free of misspelled words. It should be complete but not too wordy.

The résumé should include all vital information: your name, address, and telephone number; job objective; education and business experience. Extracurricular activities and organizations, particularly if they relate to your type of work, should also be included. For example, if you are a Certified Professional Secretary (CPS) and a member of the National Secretaries Association (NSA), be sure to list this membership. Or, if you have just finished school or college and were a member of the Future Secretaries of America, be sure to list this under the extracurricular activities section.

Because more and more women today are being placed in management positions, it would be wise to list your availability for travel and/or transfer. This could be placed under job objective on the résumé.

Under business experience, list the most recent job first. Then list your second to last job next, and so on. Be sure to list the time period involved during each employment, your immediate supervisor, the company or business name, and a brief description of your duties. For an example, see the sample résumé on page 200.

HOW TO BE PREPARED FOR THE INTERVIEW

Your whole life's destiny could be determined by the few minutes spent in an interview. For obvious reasons, you will need to be well

Résumé

MARY CAREER   Telephone Numbers:
10 Main Street   (123) 456-1234
Chicago, Illinois 12345   (123) 456-5678

JOB OBJECTIVE

I would like the opportunity to use my creative abilities
in handling routine and special events for your company.
I would like to write news releases, speeches, etc., and
perform other public relations duties. I will be available for travel and/or transfer.

EDUCATION

Highland High School, Chicago - Graduated in top 10% of
    class - 1968
University of Chicago - September, 1968 to June, 1970
    Majored in Journalism - Maintained "B" average
Northwestern University - September, 1970 to present.
    Attending evening classes. Total of 72 hours toward
    Journalism Degree. Transcript attached.
Attended special journalism seminar - San Francisco, Aug., 1971

EXTRACURRICULAR ACTIVITIES

High School - Editor of Highland Yearbook
              National Honor Society
              Cheerleader
University of Chicago - Assistant Editor of Campus Weekly News
              Member Speech Club - 1968-69
              Member National Journalism Society
Northwestern University - Member Future PR Club of America

EXPERIENCE

June, 1970 - Present   City & County Bank, Chicago
                            Half time spent in steno pool
                            Type 60 WPM; SH 100 WPM
Summer 1969   Worked in office of Chicago
                            Suburbia Newspaper. Took
                            ads over phone and did
                            general clerical work.

REFERENCES

Mr. John Doe   Mrs. Jane Jones
City and County Bank   Chicago Suburbia Newspaper
Chicago, Illinois   P. O. Box 1245
Phone (124) 666-5588   Chicago, Illinois
                            Phone (125) 423-4689

PERSONAL DATA

Age: 23 - Date of Birth: 10/10/50
Height: 5'5 1/2"   Weight: 115 lbs.
                                       Health: Excellent

prepared. The authors conducted a survey of personnel directors who interview hundreds of applicants each year. This survey revealed that a surprising number of people go into an interview partially or even totally unprepared.

Know Something about the Company. Check with your local library for sources of information on the company where you have an interview. Learn all you can about the company. You may also wish to write to the secretary of the company and request a copy of the annual report. When you know something about the organization, its history, its financial condition, the number of employees, and so on, it will not only help you, but the interviewer will be impressed that you were interested enough to find out something about the company.

Your Physical Image. The way you look and dress for the interview is more important than you may think. The initial visual image you project leaves a lasting impression; make sure it's a good one.

How should you dress for the interview? The consensus of personnel directors and interviewers in the CPI survey was as follows:

1. Be neat, clean, and well-groomed.
2. Avoid extremes in dress, makeup, hairstyle, and accessories. The girl with obviously false eyelashes, hot pants, or a see-through blouse does not project the type of image most employers want (unless he's the owner of a "go-go" club).
3. Dress as you would for the job for which you are being interviewed.
4. Do not overdress. If in doubt, dress conservatively. A bank executive very cleverly suggested that you should "look tasteful rather than tasty."
5. Demonstrate a concern for your appearance rather than an obsession with it.

If you have "thrown yourself together," it will not only be obvious to the interviewer, but you will project an image of disorganization. On the other hand, when you have thoughtfully considered every detail of your appearance, you will have increased confidence from knowing that you look your best.

Be Punctual. Arrive ahead of time for the interview. This will give you a chance to take a few deep breaths to help you relax.

If the employment application was not mailed to you before the interview, a prompt arrival will give you an opportunity to complete the form. Be sure to have your references with correct phone numbers and addresses typed out on a card in your purse. You should contact these references to ask permission before you use their names. This will also refresh their memory of you if they are contacted by your prospective employer. Also, have a copy of your school transcript in case it is requested. Answer all questions on the application form honestly and fully.

Try to anticipate questions the interviewer may ask you and be prepared to answer them truthfully and completely.

Most interviewers realize you may be nervous during the interview, but if you are well-prepared, punctual, and confident in knowing you look your best, you have fought a good fight against the battle of nerves. It may also help if you realize that this interview is not the final judgment and the interviewer is not the final judge. He is merely another person, much like yourself, trying to do a good job of placing the right person into the right job.

THE INTERVIEW

The big moment has arrived. The interviewer has just been introduced to you and you have your "foot in the door." Don't spoil your chances by blowing the interview. The survey of personnel directors and interviewers revealed some definite "do's" and "don'ts" that may be helpful. (See Figure 89.)

Interview "Do's"
1. DO let the interviewer initiate the conversation.
2. DO be relaxed and natural; be friendly but businesslike.
3. DO listen carefully and answer all questions completely and truthfully. Do not give superfluous information; answer only what is specifically asked.
4. DO be respectful and maintain good eye contact during the interview.
5. DO exhibit self-confidence. Be aware of your strengths and "sell" them. Identify your weaknesses and accept them.

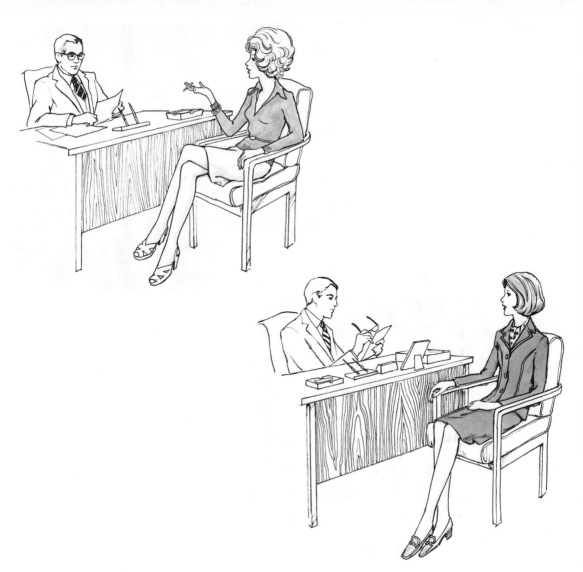

FIGURE 89.
Proper and improper ways to conduct yourself during an interview.

The word "confidence" was mentioned more than any other word by the interviewers surveyed.

Interview "Don'ts"

1. DON'T project a "Here I am! Rejoice!" attitude. Self-confidence is important but can be overdone with an arrogant attitude.
2. DON'T interview the interviewer or dominate the conversation. This is the interviewer's job, and he or she may take offense at being questioned.

3. DON'T wear sunglasses or chew gum during the interview.

4. DON'T exhibit tics and nervous habits. Biting your nails, tapping your fingers, or swinging your leg from the knee while your legs are crossed may annoy the interviewer.

5. DON'T smoke unless the interviewer is smoking and offers you a cigarette.

6. DON'T "badmouth" former employers and teachers. Be honest if questioned, and don't try to cover up anything in previous employment or scholastic history.

7. DON'T be negative about your weaknesses, but be willing to work toward improving them.

The interviewer will bring the conversation to a close at the proper time. He may do one of several things:

1. He may turn you down on the spot (in most cases an interviewer will not be this blunt).

2. He may offer you a job on the spot (if he has the authority to do this and it does not require higher approval).

3. He may arrange another interview with the proposed supervisor.

4. He may tell you he will call you if or when a decision is made.

If he turns you down, simply smile and thank him and go on to the next interview with more experience under your belt. Don't be discouraged if he tells you he will call. He may need to check with your references and compare you with the other applicants. You may still have a very good chance of getting the job. If you do not hear from him within five or six days, by all means call him inquiring about the status of the position.

Be sure to thank the person who has interviewed you. Following up with a very brief thank-you note is much appreciated by many personnel people.

In the survey, personnel directors were asked the following question: "When applicants for a particular job are narrowed down to two with similar educational and experience backgrounds, which traits, in order of importance, do you *then* consider to finalize the choice?"

The traits most often listed were as follows:

1. *Attitude*—A good attitude, a pleasant personality, and the ability to get along with others on all levels.
2. *Self-confidence*—Displaying a positive confidence in knowing you can handle the job well.
3. *Enthusiasm*—Willingness to work and having a sincere interest in the job.

An executive of a national firm told the story of an airline executive who had interviewed several men for a particular job. The applicants were finally narrowed down to Mr. "A" and Mr. "B." They had similar qualifications, but Mr. "A" had more actual job experience. However, in the final outcome, Mr. "B" was given the job simply because he wanted it more than the other applicant. He was enthusiastic about the job, and it paid off.

THE JOB

You've landed the job! You're enthusiastic, you're excited, and you've made up your mind to do your best possible work. That's great! Don't lose your enthusiasm. It will add zest to your workday as well as to your coworkers' day.

What is expected of you? Are there any rules to success?

Many companies have orientation programs to help the new employee find her way around and meet new people. At that time they often set out the particular rules for the company—the "dos" and "don'ts." These are certainly important and should be followed carefully. However, there are some "unwritten" rules of behavior that may be helpful in making your work more enjoyable, in making friends, and in helping you up the ladder of success.

Office Lifestyle. The informality that has become a way of life on the American social scene has also invaded many offices. The degree of formality depends upon the size of the office and the wishes of those in command—the boss and/or supervisor.

In response to a CPI survey, regarding the degree of formality favored in offices today, the following percentages resulted:

	Degree of Formality	Favored
Formal:	"Mr. Jones" — "Miss Smith"	7%
Semiformal:	"Mr. Jones" — "Jane"	81%
Informal:	"Jim" — "Jane"	12%

It is apparent from these statistics that the greater percentage of business executives prefer a semiformal atmosphere.

Many large offices, however, tend to be more formal not only with outsiders, but in the interpersonal relationships of the employees. On the other hand, many small offices are extremely informal.

Great care should be exercised in guarding against becoming overly familiar in your relationships with other employees in the small office. This is especially true in your relationships with the men in the office. It is best to conduct yourself in a sagacious, businesslike, and impersonal manner. Avoid becoming personally involved with those for whom you work.

Names. Always begin by calling your supervisor "Mr. Jones" or "Mrs. Brown." If they prefer being addressed by their first names, they will let you know. Even if you are on a first-name basis with your supervisor, always address him as "Mr. Jones" in the presence of a client or customer. If he is so informal that he objects, he will tell you.

You will probably call coworkers by their first names. However, if they are many years your senior, it is respectful to address them "Mrs. Brown" or "Mr. Jones" unless they specify otherwise. If you are in doubt about how to address a person, simply ask. Always address a customer or caller as "Mr. Williams" or "Miss Taylor."

Business Introductions. Regardless of your position in a company or plant, there will be times when you will be required to make introductions. Business introductions usually involve people of different ages, different sex, and different job status. Some introductions involve all of these. The person of lower rank or age is presented to the person of higher rank or age. The man is usually presented to a woman, unless she will be working for him.

The woman, the person of greater importance, or the older person's name is mentioned first. If Mr. Jones is older than Mr. Smith and you accidentally mention Mr. Smith's name first, simply add, "I would like to introduce you *to* Mr. Jones." The little word *to* corrects the error of mentioning the younger man first.

Forms of Introductions

1. Presenting a man to a woman:
   "Mrs. Brown, may I present Mr. James?"

2. Presenting a subordinate to his superior:
   "Mr. Smith, may I introduce Bill Jones?"

3. Presenting a younger person to an older person:
   "Mrs. Brown, this is Miss Young."

4. Presenting a new employee to her boss:
   "Mr. Wright, may I present Carolyn Clerk?"

5. Introducing a group such as a man and a woman meeting a woman:
   "Mrs. Brown, this is Miss Young and Mr. James."

The word "present" is a little more formal than "introduce." "This is" is informal; using nothing between the names, such as "Bill Jones, Eric James," is extremely informal.

If you should become confused while making introductions, remember that it is more important to pronounce names correctly and to clarify titles than it is to be exactly precise in your introduction etiquette.

Remembering Names. After you have met someone, it is important to remember his name. Because a person's name is usually important to him, your business success will often be enhanced if you are able to call a person by name after the first introduction. This gracious gesture of calling a client, customer, or even a coworker by name can add a plus mark toward good public relations.

A friend related the story of working with an artistically talented receptionist who would not only write down the caller's name, but would quickly sketch him on paper so that his image and name were indelibly imprinted in her mind. Other name association tricks that help jog your memory will work just as effectively.

Office Manners. The Golden Rule works just as well on the job as it does in any area of life. Doing unto others as you would want them to do unto you is such a simple rule, it is often overlooked. Good manners and everyday courtesies put the Golden Rule into action. These are essential for getting along well with your coworkers and making your work day (and theirs) enjoyable. Since you will be spending more waking hours at your job than at home, it is necessary that you enjoy your job and being with your coworkers.

Just as the physical surroundings of your office will affect your disposition, so will people. A drab and dreary room might depress you, but a bright, cheerful decor will lift your spirits. The people with whom you work will have an even greater effect on your disposition than the decor will; and you can affect their dispositions too. Be careful of your choice of words when dealing with a coworker. A curt statement, an impatient answer, or a rude reply may quickly damage an otherwise good relationship. On the other hand, you can buoy a coworker's spirit with a smile and a good disposition.

Greet your coworkers and customers cheerfully each morning— even when you would rather growl. However, don't habitually get into long conversations with your coworkers. Even if your work is up-to-date you may be interfering with theirs.

Gossip. A business executive said, "Petty gossip has no place in the business community, and yet we all—male and female—seem to thrive on it." The starting and spreading of rumors and idle gossip about coworkers or customers is a major complaint of business executives. The results of such gossip are often so widespread, they can damage or scar a person's reputation and a company's success.

One lovely career woman said she had discovered that the best way to handle gossip was to say something nice about the person in question and then quickly change the subject. It doesn't take long for the gossip to realize that you will not be a carrier of this vicious disease.

One supervisor said that, by tracing the rumor, it is often possible to find the source of the gossip. He recently heard an unusually malicious rumor about a woman employee under his supervision. The supervisor traced the rumor to a rather meek and sweet-appearing girl who finally confessed her jealousy for the woman. The supervisor suggested the girl apologize to the woman. But the piece of gossip the girl had invented had already caused irreparable damage to the woman's reputation. The supervisor fired the girl and from that time forward vowed to dismiss others who started such destructive stories.

Personal Problems. It is best to leave your personal problems out of the office. These are to be discussed only with the closest of friends, and *not* at the office.

Punctuality. Getting to the office or plant on time, but spending twenty minutes in the lounge finishing your makeup and hairdo, is really being twenty minutes late. It is a matter of professional etiquette to be on time for your job and to remain there until quitting time, except for your illness or a death or illness in your immediate family.

Lunch. Extending the lunch time beyond the alloted number of minutes will often be hard on others in your office. They may be required to answer your telephone or take care of some of your tasks while trying to do their own work. This type of behavior can damage otherwise good relationships.

Unless there is no other place provided, you should *not* eat at your desk. This is distasteful to callers as well as to coworkers.

A woman executive tells the story of going into a furniture store on her lunch hour one day. She caught the aroma of several different foods. In each department through which she walked, there were two or three employees huddled together, eating lunch on some of the coffee tables and furniture for sale. When the woman passed by the fourth such group, she finally realized that no one was going to offer to wait on her so she went to another store where she purchased a substantial amount of furniture. She was greeted immediately by a salesperson at the door of the second store. The lunch hour was still in session, but because a lunchroom had been provided for the employees of the second store, a large sale resulted.

Coffee Breaks. Coffee breaks were intended to increase the efficiency of employees by giving a fifteen-minute break from the work routine. Many employees abuse this privilege by taking too many breaks, extending the time of the breaks, and by taking them at inopportune times. For instance, a story is told about the girl who left her boss on "hold" on a long distance telephone call while she had a leisurely cup of coffee.

Telephone. Telephone manners have been discussed in Chapter Two, but it must be emphasized that you should be discreet in the use of the office or business telephone for personal calls. Our survey indicated that some women actually run their homes and children via the office telephone.

Poor Personal Habits. Someone has said that the big things in life we can take in stride, but it's the little things that get us down. So it is with poor personal habits. Listed below are some of the habits most often mentioned by business executives in the survey:

Office neatness—A sloppy desk may not bother you, but it may drive someone else crazy. Keep the office and the surroundings neat, clean, and dusted. Do not allow dirty coffee cups or unnecessary clutter to accumulate.

Excessive smoking—Some medical, dental, and business offices do not allow smoking. Abide by the rules of your particular office. If you *are* allowed to smoke, do not smoke excessively. Many people are allergic to tobacco smoke and the odor is a concern to others. When several people in a small, enclosed area smoke a great deal, a pollution problem can result.

Strong perfume, gum chewing, and *loud talking* are other personal habits frowned on by many business executives. Applying makeup or combing your hair at the desk or in public is also considered poor taste.

CONCLUSION

Regardless of whether you are a secretary, clerk, department head, or office manager, you will probably at one time or another act as an "unofficial receptionist" for your company.

If you are the first person one sees when he enters an office or a place of business, the image you project "sets the stage" for the rest of the employees and for the entire business. Therefore, the importance of projecting a *good* image cannot be overemphasized.

What is the image you project? It is the result of your attitude, appearance, speech, manner, and behavior. This image can either make or break the image of an entire place of business.

Can your image be changed? Yes, but developing a new one may involve breaking many old, annoying habits and establishing some helpful new ones. It will, however, be well worth the effort when the ultimate image you project is a good one!

ENRICHMENT ACTIVITIES

1. List the four possible ways of finding a job or arranging an interview.

2. What is a résumé?

3. Prepare a résumé on yourself with a particular prospective job in mind.

4. Prepare a letter to an interviewer inquiring about a job and asking for an appointment.

5. List several ways to be *totally* prepared for the job interview.

6. How should you dress for the interview?

7. List as many interview "dos" as you can remember. Add others *you* consider important.

8. List as many interview "don'ts" as you can remember. Add others *you* consider important.

9. What are the three traits considered most important when job applicants have been narrowed down to two?

10. Prepare a brief note to the interviewer thanking him for the appointment and interview.

11. Which is the most preferred type of office lifestyle?

    Formal _____ Semiformal _____ Informal _____

12. How do *you* feel you should address a supervisor?

13. In making simple business introductions, whose names are usually mentioned first?

14. When is a woman's name *not* mentioned first?

15. When is the little word *to* helpful in introductions?

16. Why is gossip considered to be one of the major complaints of business executives?

17. Why is projecting a good image so important?

18. List some poor personal habits.

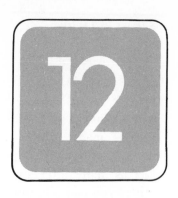

you and your
life style

Severing the invisible umbilical cord that binds you to home is a big step. The day comes when you decide you are ready to set out on your own, get a job, and develop your own lifestyle (Figure 90). Yes, your own lifestyle—when you can truly become *you*—to experience, taste, express, feel, think, decide, yearn . . . all the countless expressions that well up from that inner core of Self. You are going to make mistakes, no doubt about it. You are going to become angry at *you* for stupidity and carelessness, but you're going to *learn*. This chapter is designed to help you avoid some of the pitfalls of living on your own so that you can develop your lifestyle with relative comfort and ease.

SELECTING AND LOCATING THE APARTMENT

When you make your big move, possibly to a city, you have two important goals: First, find a job, then find a place to live. These are the things you must do before you can settle into the adventure of living, working, and having fun in the city.

You must have enough money to see you through one month of getting settled. The following expenses should be considered during the first month of The Great Change: transportation; meals; temporary living; miscellaneous expenses such as entertainment, snacks, and cokes; cleaning and laundry; and the hairdresser. Should you

212

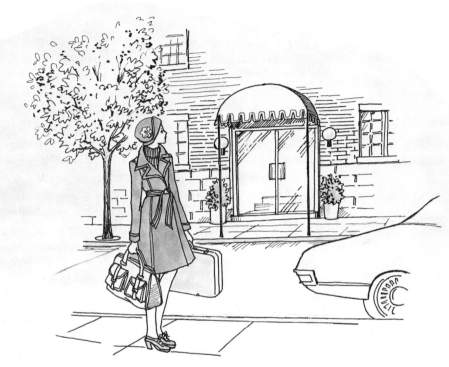

FIGURE 90.
Severing the invisible umbilical cord that binds you to home is a big step.

take an apartment immediately, you must be prepared to pay the first month's rent in advance plus a deposit for damages. You will have to pay a deposit for a phone and, perhaps, other utilities. Allowing some extra dollars for getting basically settled into an apartment, or for an emergency fund, it is safe to say that you'll need a considerable nest egg!

It is advisable to find your job *first*; then locate your living quarters. Transportation to and from work, such as freeways, bus service, or subway, should be carefully examined. As one apartment locator expressed, "It is very unfortunate to find an apartment for a girl and then have her take a job many miles from where she lives." The job's location may determine where you will want to live.

If you are fortunate in being close to your chosen city or town, then, ideally, you can locate your job and apartment without making a temporary move. Another alternative is to stay with friends or relatives. If you do this, don't expect a free ride, particularly with single girls on tight salaries. Put something in the pot for groceries. Don't expect them to "wine and dine" you. After all, they are accommodating you. If you are using someone's car, then chip in on the gas, and if you use it a great deal, you might show your appreciation by having it washed. Above all, be a thoughtful guest and offer to help around the house or apartment.

The third solution for the truly independent person, and the most economical, is to stay at the YWCA until you are settled; however, do call ahead to make a reservation and learn the various rates and requirements. They vary slightly depending on the locale.

Unless you are familiar with your chosen city, you will be wise to secure the assistance of an apartment locator service. There is often no charge for helping you find an apartment because the fee is paid by the apartment owner. The service will provide you with a list of available apartments suitable for your needs. If you do not know your way around, some services will even drive you to the apartments. This is a tremendous advantage and a sure timesaver when so many apartments are readily available and are using glamorous advertising campaigns. In choosing an apartment, think about the following: the rent, management and maintenance; general atmosphere, size and layout of the apartment; conveniences, such as laundry facilities and parking; special facilities such as pool, game room, garden, patio, and so on; and whether it is well-located in relation to work, shopping centers, and desirable neighbors.

When you rent an apartment, you may have to sign a lease agreement. Read it! It will detail your privileges, the apartment rules and regulations, maintenance and repairs, pet restrictions, and utility payments. It is important to find out how binding the lease agreement is in the event of a job transfer or marriage. Certainly there are unavoidable circumstances, but in some areas, landlords, wearied of the fickle singles' propensity for apartment-hopping, have toughened up on leases. As mentioned before, you will have to pay a damage deposit, which should be returned to you when you leave, provided no damage has been done. If you have a pet, some apartments require a separate deposit for *each* animal. Stay away from pets until you can afford them. Besides the pet deposit, the cost of food, vet charges, and your time make a pet a luxury you can't afford.

SHARING THE APARTMENT

Sharing the apartment with one or more girls cuts down on expenses, provides one with companionship, and makes those early days of starting out on your own much easier. It's nice to have "roomies" to shares those boo-boos you make at work or your excitement at meeting that special man. Having and sharing your own apartment in no way compares to living at home or in a dorm. You will learn the give-and-take business of living together. To be a happy experience, it must be based on cooperation, consideration, respect, and responsibility. Sounds a bit like marriage, doesn't it?

There's no yardstick for picking a roommate. Frequently it just happens through ex-school friends, work, church, or mutual friends. There are roommate referral services. Sometimes your best friend may not be the best roommate for you, or you for her. It is important to find someone who has attitudes, ideas, interests, and morals compatible with yours. Here are a few suggestions that might lead to harmonious roommating:

1. Do sit down and decide how you and your roommate (or roommates) are going to handle money matters and household responsibilities. You will also have to work together on decorating and furnishing the apartment.

2. You will have to decide how you will handle the groceries and meals. This can be done in several ways, depending on your individual situation.

   a. When there are only two roommates, some girls prefer to buy such things as staples, perishables, and household cleaning items together and shop for themselves separately. This works for girls who are, for instance, dieting or dating frequently.

   b. Some prefer a "kitty," putting in equal portions a month and sharing most of the meals together.

   c. When there are four or more, storage is a problem if everyone has her own supply, so a kitty works better in this situation.

   d. If you plan to have a guest over for dinner, then put something extra in the kitty or shop for it separately.

   e. You may want to add a little extra to the kitty for newspaper subscriptions.

3. Handle the phone bill fairly. Do not agree to split the total amount, unless you want to pay for long distance calls that are not your own.

4. Purchase household items individually so that when you

break up housekeeping it is not a problem as to *who* owns *what*.

5. You should decide on a routine of duties and they should be rotated. You may decide to take turns cooking or cleaning. You may divide the apartment up into different areas to clean. Above all, the duties must be distributed, rotated, and shared fairly. It is very important that each roommate have the responsibility of grocery shopping and paying the rent and utility bills. This is good experience for the future.

6. Be fair about entertaining in the apartment. Don't monopolize the television and living room. You might try keeping a calendar of your activities. Although you want to feel free and independent, it is simple consideration to let your roommate know something of your plans. If you plan to be gone overnight, you should let her know. This could be for your own protection.

7. Be loyal to your roommate and courteous to her friends. Don't flirt with her men. Be kind to her relatives. Be understanding. And accept each other's individuality.

Decorating and furnishing the apartment must be agreeable to all roommates. It may be cheaper to rent a furnished apartment until you have acquired enough furniture to move into an unfurnished one. However, there are many inexpensive "do-it-yourself" routes that you can take. Thus, it seems a shame to rent furniture. With imagination, ingenuity, and patience you can create an apartment that is homey, chic, sophisticated, cute . . . at most, a reflection of *your* personality and life style.

Forget about buying a bedroom suite. Taste can change as a person matures, and it is best not to restrict yourself too early to furniture suites. Buy a single bed that can serve as a couch, guest bed, or a bed for "Junior" in the future. You are not limited by a particular period and can change easily. Headboards can range from wicker, purchased at import stores, to mantels, shelves, and brass headboards from antique stores; or try a wild array of pillows.

Storage is always a problem in an apartment, and a good chest is essential. Unpainted chests can be antiqued, covered with adhesive paper, or painted a bright, contemporary color. Many used-furniture stores and antique stores have old chests, but unless they are in good condition and the drawers pull easily, you are wise to invest in an unpainted one.

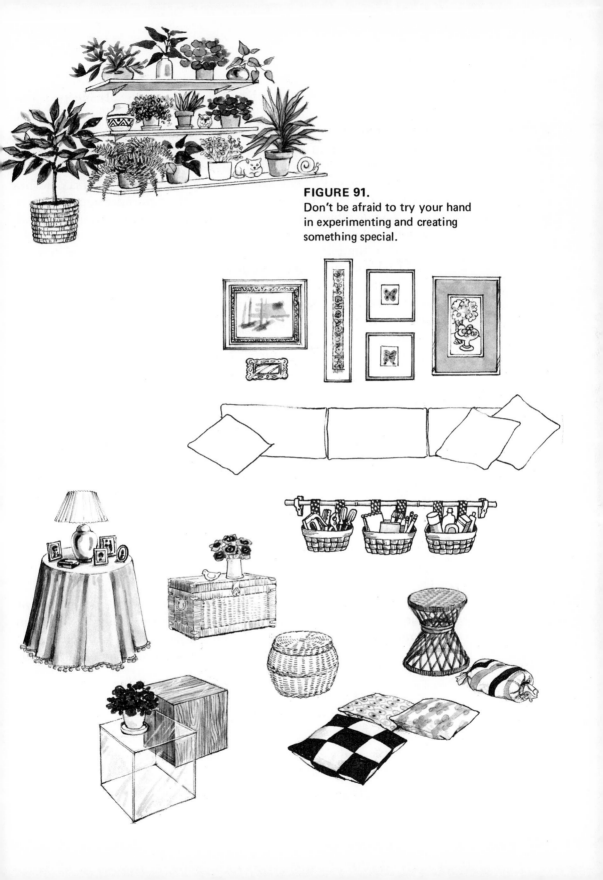

FIGURE 91.
Don't be afraid to try your hand
in experimenting and creating
something special.

An elegant dressing table can be made by placing two low, unpainted chests side by side, leaving enough space for your knees, and topping them with either fake marble or glass. From import stores and South of the Border, baskets can be purchased at nominal prices. These baskets can function not only as decorative items but for storage as well. They can serve as magazine baskets, dirty clothes hampers, or coffee tables, depending on the size and shape.

Round tables with pretty, long cloths seem to fit every mood, period, and style. Some stores offer unfinished bases and round tops that serve the purpose inexpensively. Unfinished cubes, which make clever tables, can also be antiqued, painted, or covered.

If you want a collection of pictures and can't afford it, learn to make your own frames, both plaster of Paris and wood. Collect pictures from greeting cards, wallpaper, gift wrapping paper, and magazines. Learn the art of découpage, and you can have an interesting collage of pictures to place over the couch or on a drab wall.

Greenery is a must. There is something about green plants in an apartment that creates both a "homey" and sophisticated atmosphere. Try an arrangement of plants in a window, or on a row of shelves—anywhere will work. Paint clay pots a sparkling white. Mix your live plants with fake ones and create your own "forest primeval." Study magazines and newspapers for decorating tips. Visit department stores and arts and crafts shops. Don't be afraid to experiment and try your hand in creating something (Figure 91).

HANDLING THE "BIG BUSINESS"

Once you get the beautiful paycheck, you're going to have to determine how to spend it. For at least three months, keep track of your expenses. Keep these in a simple journal so that you can get an overall picture of where your money is going. A budget is an individual thing; however, the following items are the most typical:

> Apartment rent
> Food and beverages
> Phone
> Gas and electricity (usually included in apartment rent)
> Laundry and dry cleaning
> Drugs and cosmetics

> Car payment and maintenance (or transportation)
> Clothes
> Insurance (medical, car, household)
> Hairdresser
> Dental and doctor bills
> Furniture
> Entertainment
> Miscellaneous (gifts, donations)

There is a lot for that paycheck to cover, and it will only stretch so far. Here are a few rules that might help you cope with the problem of "high finance."

1. Use castoffs from home. Scrounge for old pots, pans, and dishes. Remember you are not a bride.
2. Save your trading stamps to buy new things for your apartment.
3. Don't pay too much for your apartment. Be patient in developing your lifestyle.
4. As mentioned before, be patient, too, with your decorating impulses.
5. The hairdresser can be a big expense; learn to do your hair, wig, and hairpieces yourself.
6. Be a thoughtful, generous friend, but don't go in debt for gifts, especially at Christmas.
7. Remember that long distance phone calls can add up.
8. Beware of the salesman who comes knocking at your door to sell you some fantastic cookware.
9. All girls love clothes. Do plan and coordinate your wardrobe rather than buying haphazardly. Buy clothes that fit your way of life, and use discipline with apparel you don't need.
10. Study newspaper ads for bargains in both wearing apparel and grocery items. Incidentally, avoid shopping in the grocery store every day or grabbing items at convenient stores where the prices are higher.

Another decision you must make in the world of high finance is selecting your bank. When you open your checking account, you should choose a bank based on the following:

1. Convenience—both in location and in banking hours.
2. Personnel—the friendliness and helpfulness of the banking staff.
3. The stability of the bank.
4. Service charge or maintenance fee—banks vary on this; investigate before opening your account.

Writing checks and keeping your checkbook balanced is your responsibility. It is never very pleasant, but a few rules can keep it from being too painful.

1. Sign your checks just as you signed your signature card when you first opened your account.
2. Write your checks carefully. Keep a record of each one. Do it the minute you write out your check. Never write a check in pencil as it is too easy to change. Never leave spaces where words or figures can be added. Do not make out your check to "cash" and sign it, as anyone can cash it. Endorse your checks with your signature and "for deposit only" written on the back. Bring your balance forward each time you write a check. This is one way to avoid being overdrawn.

Make a habit of balancing your books every month. Either have your bank statement mailed or pick it up each month and then reconcile your statement. It really does not require a course in bookkeeping to do so. First, put your checks in order by their number. Check the ones that have come in. Write down the last balance shown on the bank statement. Write down any deposits you've made since the date of the statement. Add the last balance and the deposits together. List any outstanding checks (those listed but not included in your statement), and total these checks. Subtract the service fee (which will be shown on the front of the statement) from *your checkbook* balance. Your reconciled balance is thus obtained by subtracting your outstanding checks from the total of your last balance and the deposits that were not shown on your statement. Most statements have a form on the back similar to the example illustrated in Figure 92.

You will need to establish credit. Most stores will ask for a driver's license and a credit card when cashing checks. A gas credit card is good to have with you, not only for identification but for security in traveling. Charge accounts are helpful, especially at Christmas, but avoid having too many or overcharging. Once you have a bad credit rating, it takes five to seven years to reestablish it. You do have access to your credit rating record at local credit bureaus. Periodically check to see that it is in order.

Developing your lifestyle means assuming the problems and responsibilities of an independent person as well as having fun. It means taking the time to organize your business affairs, even if you have to say "no" to a social occasion. It means developing a system of organization. Don't be like the girl who turns her bedroom into a disaster area every time she needs a certain paper. Create a filing system, even if it is in an old shoe box; of course, a metal lock box will offer more security. Keep your *cancelled checks*. This is very important not only for tax purposes, but for the time when you need to prove that you paid a bill. Keep your checks for at least two years. Keep your *bank statements, check stubs*, and *deposit slips*. Keep

FIGURE 92.
Make a habit of balancing your books every month.

BANK STATEMENT

1. Bank balance shown on statement————
2. Plus (if any) deposits not on statement————
3. Add items 1 and 2. Showing total here ————
4. List outstanding checks below. ————
5. Minus (if any) outstanding checks————
6. Your reconciled balance should agree
   with your checkbook balance————

Outstanding checks	
No.	Amount
Total	

sales slips until you are satisfied with the merchandise. Keep your *social security card, tax returns, car title, voter registration, birth certificate, insurance policies*, and *contracts* in an organized manner.

PURCHASING A CAR

One of the biggest investments that you will make will be in a car—that is, if you didn't receive one gratis. Nevertheless, you still have the responsibility of protecting that investment. The following are some tips on car financing as well as car maintenance.

As has been previously advised, you should establish credit at the bank of your choice. Your bank will assist you in choosing a reputable automobile dealer.

The most important thing in the purchase of an automobile is the financing. Finance the purchase through your bank where you have established credit. Bank finance charges are usually less on new and used cars than those of finance companies. Insurance requirements on bank financing are also better because the bank does not require a specific insurance agent or company and will require only the necessary insurance to protect their loan. Most cars are financed over a three-year period. However, your insurance policy with bank financing will be written on a yearly basis. The financing of an automobile is very often the beginner's downfall. The importance of checking this carefully cannot be stressed enough.

After making the purchase, your thoughts should turn to selecting a service station for the care of your car. It is important to choose a station that is convenient to your residence and on your way to work. Remember, there is a difference between a service station and a *filling* station: A filling station operator will fill your tank; a *service* station operator will service your car. The one you select should take an interest in your car. Many maintain a file on customers' cars and will remind you when you need an oil change (about every 3,000 miles, depending on the car), when you should have your filter changed, when you should have wheel bearings checked (10,000 miles), when you should have your transmission checked, and when the tires should be checked. Never authorize car repairs without *first* obtaining an estimate of parts and labor. Careful attention to the preceding items by both you and your service station attendant will mean a smooth-running vehicle and a savings on repair bills, which could cost you a staggering amount.

Other personal obligations you will encounter will be insurance and hospitalization. Before signing any dotted lines, seek counsel from people whose knowledge you respect; in fact, the only way you will learn to handle business affairs is by asking questions and by relying on the advice of more experienced people.

PROTECTING YOURSELF

There are a number of common-sense safety precautions that you should make as much a habit of your daily life as brushing your teeth. Although there's no guarantee in life, every woman owes it to herself to take the steps that will ensure her every possible margin of safety, whether she is married or single, from a small town or the city. The following do's and don'ts will serve as an insurance policy against possible unpleasantness.

1. When you move into your apartment, change your locks (if permitted by your apartment manager). Have only a certain number of keys made up for each roommate and an extra for any overnight guest. Don't let this "guest key" escape you.
2. Make a habit of carrying your key and keeping it with you. Before you leave for work or a date, check and double-check your purse for your key. It's no fun being locked out of your own apartment. Keep your house key on a separate chain, not with your car keys.
3. Don't leave extra keys in mailboxes or under the doormat. And above all, don't leave notes that say, "Dear Jane, the key is under the pot plant" unless you like to extend engraved invitations to prowlers.
4. When you leave the apartment, if only to empty the trash, lock the door. Lock it even if your roommates are at home. Someone could slip in while you are gone.
5. Be sure you have a chain guard and a double lock or dead bolt for all outside doors. For sliding glass doors, a broom or mop handle placed in the treads will prevent anyone from opening it.
6. Be dressed or properly robed when you answer the door.
7. *Don't let strangers into your apartment.* If your apartment doesn't have a peephole, ask your apartment manager if you may install one. Never take the chain guard off when

you answer the door. If someone is collecting money, for donations or a newspaper for example, and you must leave to get the money, close and *lock the door behind you*. If a stranger needs to borrow the phone, offer to make the call for him, but *lock the door behind you*. Certainly we like to be good Samaritans, but the tragedy today is that too many trusting, good Samaritans get hurt. Always verify maintenance and repair men by checking with the manager or requiring identification.

8. Don't hesitate to leave a light burning at the front and back entrance if you plan to return after dark; it's worth the few cents to ensure your safety. Timers can be installed that will automatically turn on your lights. A television or radio left playing will act as a deterrent against a prowler.

9. Most apartments have outside mailboxes. A slot is provided for the name of the apartment dweller. Don't advertise that you are a single girl—just use your initial and last name. The same rule applies to listing your name in the telephone book.

10. Do not be liberal with information over the phone; *ask* questions of the person calling rather than *answering* his questions.

11. Always have a companion when you use the laundry room late at night.

12. When you travel in the car, keep your doors locked day and night. If possible, avoid traveling alone at night. Always keep your gas tank filled rather than running the risk of being caught without gas on some lonely road. If you must travel at night, stay on the main streets and park in well-lighted areas. Before entering your car, look into the back seat. Lock your car when you leave it; when you approach it, have your keys out and ready. Keep a flashlight in your car. If you have car trouble on a highway, tie a white handkerchief to the antenna, put the hood up, and lock yourself inside the car. Wait for the police to help you. Do not go off with strangers!

13. Leave your garage light on if you plan to return home after dark.

14. If you are on foot at night, walk briskly and in well-lighted areas. Don't hesitate to report suspicious strangers.

ENTERTAINING ON A BUDGET

Entertaining in your own home can be fun and excellent experience for the future; however, unless it is planned carefully, it can be a drain and strain on your pocketbook. The key to entertaining on a budget is *planning*. Decide your menu based on your own knowledge, time, and money. An old saying goes, "The way to a man's heart is through his stomach." Consequently, it is wiser to experiment on your girlfriends than on your boyfriends. Don't plan a dinner that will keep you in the kitchen the entire evening. Make your shopping list carefully so that you arrive home from the grocery store with all the essential items. Check your own supplies so that you don't buy unnecessarily. Make a list of all the things you will have to do for the evening. Avoid elaborate meals and costly food items. Don't skimp on the quantity of food! Learn to be a gracious hostess and, most of all, laugh rather than cry at your mistakes.

TAKING THE CULTURAL ROUTE

Developing your lifestyle encompasses all the broad aspects of life: not only the responsibilities, but also those aspects that will enrich your life. Those who are fortunate enough to live in or near a city should take advantage of all the opportunities it has to offer, but don't write off the small town as a cultural desert. Explore all the possibilities your location has to offer you. Though your budget is limited, there are many free educational and cultural avenues open. For example, the library, although once merely a place to check out books, now offers many services to its community. Museums and art galleries enable an individual to learn about the art of many periods—from the old masters to contemporary painters and sculptors. Throughout the country, many cities are offering free theater, such as Houston's Miller Theater, where people see such lavish productions as *South Pacific* and *Gypsy*. Community theaters provide you with the chance to involve yourself personally.

COMMUNITY INVOLVEMENT

Personal involvement does not have to be cultural or educational. It could be offering your services to your community. People are needed to work with youth groups, senior citizens, the underprivileged, and in hospitals. Newspaper columns are printed weekly, listing various volunteer jobs open.

Take the time to read your local newspaper. It will keep you abreast of what is happening around town. As you take different avenues of life, you will learn more about yourself, your own interests and tastes, and you will truly develop your individual lifestyle.

ENRICHMENT ACTIVITIES

1. Write to the YWCA in the city of your choice to find out information regarding rates and requirements.
2. Study want ads for apartments in your locale.
3. Make a "housekeeping notebook." Include a list of all necessities for establishing apartment living, the household duties, and an inexpensive decor.
4. Familiarize yourself with the costs of individual grocery items.
5. Plan several inexpensive meals for entertaining.
6. Write to the Chamber of Commerce of your chosen city for information on employment, entertainment, and transit services.
7. Visit an art museum or gallery. Make a list of the artists whose work you admired.
8. Using your newspaper's entertainment section, list all cultural activities available during a month's time.
9. Secure a booklet entitled "Personal Money Management" published by The American Bankers' Association. Percentage figures have been compiled as a guide for establishing a budget. Devise your own budget using a typical salary.
10. List the volunteer jobs printed in your newspaper.

what every woman should know about the law

ALIMONY—BRIDGE OVER TROUBLED WATERS

In some states it is called *support* and in others it is called *maintenance*, but it adds up to the same thing: the obligation that continues after divorce to support the wife, and it is usually called *alimony*. The court can grant alimony from the beginning of divorce proceedings. In some states this is called *temporary alimony* and in other states *alimony pendente lite*.

Most states have adopted the "no fault" approach to divorce. In the past, the court heard much evidence as to who caused the marital breakup. Now the issue is whether the marriage can or cannot be salvaged. Having determined that it cannot, the court grants a divorce.

Alimony is granted or not by the court, depending on the circumstances of the wife. If she is able to take care of herself, the court may not grant alimony. If the husband is not able to take care of himself, the court may order the wife to pay alimony. Those cases, however, usually make headlines.

The judge determines the amount of alimony, based on the facts presented to him. As the facts change, so does the amount of alimony. If alimony is fixed at a time when the husband has a low

227

salary and he subsequently becomes a highly-paid executive, the court can increase the alimony. On the other hand, if he goes from riches to rags, the court can and will take that circumstance into account in reducing the alimony.

Usually, it is best for parties contemplating divorce to arrange their own agreement concerning alimony and to obtain the approval of the court on the decision they have made. This saves the time, trouble, and anguish of a court proceeding, and if the parties are realistic about the outcome of the hearing, they will agree in advance to an amount of alimony.

Thus, after the marital tie is severed, alimony continues.

BAIL—FREEDOM UNTIL TRIAL

Bail is a system devised under our law to prevent a person from being punished before his guilt has been established. A person accused of crime is given temporary freedom after putting up a sum of money, usually substantial, to guarantee his appearance in court when his case is to be heard.

Almost every accused person is entitled to get out of jail on bail. The exceptions have been cases known as "capital crimes" in which the evidence against the person charged with the crime is particularly strong. "Capital crime" is one by which the death penalty could be assessed, and the theory is that anyone who is faced with the possibility of the death penalty would be tempted to flee the country or go into hiding rather than be on hand for the trial. Most persons charged with a crime do go free on bail. Most of those who remain in prison are entitled to bail but cannot afford it.

Who sets the bail, and how high should it be? The Constitution (Eighth Amendment) requires that bail not be excessive. The way bail is determined in each case involves many factors. One of those is whether the accused has ever jumped bail before. High bail may be set for him because he could be expected to do it again. Bail should be set higher for a felony charge than for a misdemeanor.

The rights of poor people have come before the courts in recent years. When it has been shown that even the smallest bail could not be raised by the accused, it has been argued that he is being required to remain in jail because of his poverty. Bail reforms have been undertaken in most places, and bail is not required for the indigent defendant who, on a case-by-case basis, gives evidence that he will be on hand when his case comes to trial. In setting bail, the judge takes into account whether the accused has a family, job, residence, ties with the town, and other indications of stability.

The accused is presumed to be innocent until he is proven guilty. If he can be released, with reasonable safety to society, then society is relieved of the necessity of confining him and bearing the cost of keeping him until his day in court.

CHILDREN—RESPONSIBILITY FOR LITTLE VISITORS

When children come to your home for a visit, you expect to treat them with hospitality. The law imposes something more on you, however: that you use every reasonable means of providing for their safety. If you fail in this, you can be legally responsible if the little visitor is hurt.

Freddie, age nine, and his brother, age six, came to your house to swing. Freddie was on the swing with you giving him a push, but you failed to notice that his little brother was walking in front of the swing. The inevitable happened, and the little brother was knocked down and hurt. Are you liable? Yes, you may be. Because of the tender age of the little brother, you should have been on the lookout for unexpected things he might do.

You can be held liable for damages for failing to do something. Assume that you would not let your six-year-old play on the second-story balcony because the railing was inadequate but you permitted the six-year-old child next door to do so. In the event of injury, the court might hold you liable on the theory that you owed as much duty to the neighbor child as you did to your own.

On the other hand, accidents can be accidents and no one is to blame. Where you could not foresee that the condition was dangerous, you would be free from liability.

DIVORCE—DIVISION OF THE PROGENY

Divorce divides not only man and wife but often splits the children. One of the most difficult functions of the divorce court is the exercise of its power to grant the children to the mother or the father, or to separate them. There is a presumption that each spouse is a fit parent and one has no greater claim to the children than the other. No matter what is good for the divided parents, the court is usually very reluctant to separate the children because it knows that it is better for children to be with each other. That is why, in most divorce cases, one parent gets the custody of all the children.

On the other hand, in some cases it is better to separate the children than to keep them together. When one is a delinquent and the other is not, the court might decide that it is certainly better to separate the children, recognizing that the children learn much—good and bad—from each other.

What does the court do about age and sex of children concerning their custody? In the child's best interests, the court could decide that the girl should live with the mother and the boy should live with the father on the assumption that the boy needs the discipline of a father.

The father can often provide greater financial security than the mother. Does the court give much weight to this in awarding children to fathers in a divorce case? The answer is no. Even though the father could provide more material goods and things of pleasure, the court's concern for the welfare of the children usually is centered most on the emotional and intellectual growth and development of the children than on material things.

ESTATE PLANNING—LIVE AND DIE WITH PROBATE

Did you know that everybody has a "will"? If you haven't prepared one yourself, the state in which you live prepared one for you, generally referred to as the law of inheritance or the statute of descent and distribution. If you fail to make a will, the state draws up a plan to dispose of your property at your death. You may wonder how the state knows what you want to do with your property. The answer is that, in the judgment of legislators years ago, the "average" person would want to dispose of his property in a certain way, and they figure that you are average.

Pretty good theory, but it often has bad results. Consider the case of the man who had two children—a son who was a ne'er-do-well and a daughter who stayed home and took care of him. The father helped the daughter go into business but the business was unsuccessful and she lost the $10,000 he gave her. The father died without a will. Everyone knew he intended to cut off the ne'er-do-well son and leave his estate to his daughter; but under the laws of inheritance of his state, his son got $10,000 from the state first to equalize what the daughter had received, and then shared half of everything with her.

One of the other cruel effects of dying without a will is the effect on a small estate. In most places the widow gets only part of the estate, but many men think the widow gets the whole estate and, thus, they do not make a will. If there are children, the children inherit a portion of the estate; but because they are small, they can't receive it, and the law provides that the estate must be tied up until the children become of legal age or are otherwise declared adults. This results in years of court costs, attorneys' fees, and trouble.

Another thing wrong with the "will" that the state makes for a person who does not make a will for himself is that such a will makes no provision for those outside the family you might like to remember, such as church, school, or charity. Nor does it make provision for a gift to dear friends. Every person should have a lawyer-drawn will.

FOOD AND DRUG LAWS—PUBLIC PROTECTION

Who does not recall the tragedy of the thalidomide babies, those born deformed? A drug was used before it had been thoroughly tested. Who protects the public? The Food and Drug Administration is a government bureau established to regulate research and development of new products to make sure they can be used without harm.

Every day new drugs are developed. Old diseases give way to new treatments. Manufacturers make extensive investments as they produce new drugs. The cost of drugs today reflects how much is spent for research and development. The actual cost of producing the drugs we take is only a fraction of the price we pay; the difference, in part, is the cost of developing other drugs.

If you take a drug prescribed by a physician and it produces a serious side effect, can the manufacturer be liable? Indeed he can. These cases are generally referred to as "product liability" cases, and every day courts across the nation award large judgments for damages people suffer as the result of unexpected side effects.

The other responsibility of the Food and Drug Administration is food. It is never-ending process to make sure that sellers sell and buyers consume pure food. Those who knowingly sell contaminated food not only can be liable for civil damages but can be punished for criminal violations of the law.

Foreign matter in food is another source of litigation. For example, a customer in a cafe was injured by a stone in a serving of peas, and the court held the restaurant liable because it felt that when a customer is served food, he can reasonably expect that it is free of stones and should be able to rely on those preparing the food to remove foreign substances from whatever the customer is being offered to eat.

GUNS—RIGHT (AND LIABILITY) TO BEAR ARMS

One of the most tragic accidents involves a gun and a child. Each year a leading cause of death or injury is a gun fired by a child. It is well known that children do not know how to handle guns and often shoot or are shot by loaded guns left within their reach. A typical case is that of an eleven-year-old boy and his chum playing after school before the mother came home from work. His mother kept a gun for household protection, and he knew where it was located. He and his chum were playing with the gun and five minutes before his mother came home from work, his chum was dead.

The laws of all states make it a criminal offense for anyone to give or sell a gun to a minor under a certain age, often seventeen years of age. The courts of many states will hold the owner of the gun liable for damage or injury done with it by a child, regardless of how careful the adult is. Ordinarily, a parent is not liable for legal wrongs his child commits, but he may be held liable by the courts if his child obtains a gun that causes injury to another person.

Guns seem to be an "attractive nuisance" to a child. It is common knowledge that children, particularly boys, engage in imaginary shooting matches with their friends. The courts have found that boys are generally eager to possess and use guns, and those who allow immature children to possess a gun can be held responsible. Anyone who owns a gun and allows a child to use it will be held liable if someone is thereby injured.

The right to bear arms is a privilege, similar to the right to drive an automobile, and each state can require a resident to obtain a license before acquiring a gun. The license, once granted, can be revoked if the person holding it fails to maintain a high standard of responsibility.

HOMICIDE—EXCUSED OR PUNISHED

If a person is driving his car carefully and another person dashes in front of his car and is killed, it is homicide. If a person is driving the same automobile at a high rate of speed, weaving in and out of traffic, and a person dashes across his path and is killed, this too, is homicide. Which is excused and which is punished? Of course, the former is excused and the latter is not. If the death is not the result of criminal negligence, it is not a crime. Today, with so many automobile accidents, this type of homicide is a frequent occurrence. If an assailant attacks you and you defend yourself from his attack and kill him, the courts hold that this is justifiable homicide.

Death in the prize fight ring is another instance of homicide. If the fight is approved by the legal authorities, the survivor would not be guilty of a crime; but if not licensed, the reverse would be true.

Can you kill in defense of your property? This is a more difficult question. To take a human life in defense of property, you must show that there was an emergency, that you gave warning, or that you were not able to give warning, that you used reasonable caution, and that there was no intention to cause the death.

In some states one who kills another while engaged in a criminal offense, even though he did not intend to kill, will be held criminally liable.

Generally, the test to determine whether you would be justfied in killing in self-defense are: (1) you must be in imminent danger of death or bodily harm if you do not act, (2) the danger must seem to be real at the time, (3) some states say that you must retreat rather than kill, and (4) you must not have provoked the attack or been the aggressor.

An example of justifiable homicide is a woman who kills to protect herself from assault.

INSANITY—A STATE OF MIND

There is no hard and fast definition for insanity. *Sane* and *insane* are relative terms, and there is a considerable gray area in between.

From time immemorial the criminal law has required that to be punished, a person committing a crime must have an "evil mind." In criminal law an insane person cannot have an evil mind and, thus, is not punished for crimes he commits but is rather committed for medical treatment.

On the other hand, an insane person cannot escape liability for civil damages and wrongs. The law has reasoned that it is better for the wrong-doer's assets to be used to compensate his victim than to have the victim suffer no recompense.

When a person is insane, he may need a guardian because he cannot transact business for himself. If the person has a spouse who is not disqualified, that spouse is entitled to be appointed his guardian in preference to any other person. If he has no spouse, then his children have that right. If he has no children, other kindred in the order set forth in the law can act for him.

According to eminent psychiatrists, nobody is perfectly sane.

JURY SERVICE—PRICE OF DEMOCRACY

Trial by jury has come down to us through the centuries as a part of the English-American tradition. It is slow, costly, and often regarded as inefficient; but no system has ever been devised to take its place.

Jurors are selected for civil cases and criminal cases in a similar manner. Names are usually drawn by lot, and persons called for jury service are known as *veniremen*. A *grand* jury is an investigative body, and a *petit* jury is the trial jury. The laws in most states exempt certain people from jury duty, usually teachers, mothers who have children, and old and infirm persons.

A jury is usually made of twelve persons, although six persons are used in some lower courts. In some states alternate jurors are picked for jury duty to take the place of any juror who becomes ill. An alternate juror does not take part in the jury discussion or vote unless called upon to replace one of the regular jurors who becomes ill, disabled, or is dismissed. When a venireman's name is called by the clerk of the court, he or she takes a seat in the jury box. The attorneys, or sometimes the judge, give a brief outline of the case and the veniremen are questioned by the attorneys and the judge. This questioning is referred to as *voir dire*. A prospective juror is asked questions to see if he has any connection with the case or has any prejudice against the parties, the attorneys, or the judge. If he does, the juror may be dismissed from the jury panel. An example of good causes for challenging a juror is prejudice with respect to insurance. It is fairly common knowledge that most jurors tend to rule against insurance companies and for the working man. On the other hand, people who work for insurance companies tend to favor the insurance company over the working man.

The attorneys in the case have a right to reject a certain number of prospective jurors without any reason whatsoever, called "peremptory challenges." This allows a lawyer to dismiss a venireman because the lawyer has a hunch that the juror would not be favorable to his side of the case but is without evidence on which to base that hunch.

After the full number of jurors has been selected, the case goes to trial. Sometimes the selection of a jury takes a considerable amount of time.

Notwithstanding its shortcomings, the jury system has proved its worth and when one is called for jury service, he or she should regard the call as an opportunity to pay, in a small way, the price of democracy.

LANDLORDS AND TENANTS—RENT CHECKS AND WATER PIPES

Usually the person who is in control of a building is the only one liable for its defective condition. If the tenant has control, he is liable. This is true of an apartment, store, theater, and so forth. If you fall and are injured as a result of a defect in the floor of the store, is the operator the only one responsible to you, or can the owner of the building be held liable? Often this makes the difference between being paid for an injury or not. The store operator may have little in the way of assets and perhaps no insurance, but the owner of the building may be a person of substantial means.

It is the usual rule that when the owner of a building turns over possession and control of it to someone else, he is not responsible to anyone else after the tenant takes possession. An exception is in the case of a concealed defect in the premises. The law of most states requires the owner of the building to inspect it and put it in suitable condition before he turns over its possession to his tenant. The landlord can be held liable on the theory that he knows his property best and should not be allowed to shift responsibility to his tenant if, by making repairs, he could prevent danger to others. The liability of the owner of the building is particularly great when the property is to be used by the public, as distinguished from private residences.

The landlord's liability is not limited to paying customers but includes anyone lawfully on the premises. Persons who come to a store, whether they purchase or not, are covered by the landlord's obligation. Likewise, social visitors enjoy that same protection.

A landlord has certain rights concerning property he rents. He may reserve the right to inspect the premises himself for repairs.

Of course, if a tenant violates his rental agreement or lease, he may be dispossessed by court order.

When the lease expires, the owner of the premises can expect it to be returned to him in as good condition as when it was leased, except for ordinary wear and tear.

MARRIAGE—FOR BETTER FOR WORSE

George Bernard Shaw, that Irish wit, said that "marriage is popular because it combines the maximum of temptation with the maximum of opportunity."

Marriage is a great deal more than sex. It is a great deal more than a private agreement. The state in which the ceremony is performed is a party to every marriage contract.

A promise to marry is a contract, and refusal to keep the promise is a breach of contract. "Heart balm" lawsuits were once popular, and many of them were filed all across the nation. Now many states have abolished breach-of-contract-to-marry cases because they have often been found to be false and fraudulent claims.

Marriage laws vary from state to state, but in all states certain similar requirements can be found. The age at which a person can marry is one of them. In most states the minimum age for marriage is eighteen years for males and sixteen years for females, but these rules differ from state to state, particularly when the birth of a child is imminent.

Common-law marriage is a legally binding arrangement without marriage license or the formal ceremony. It is based on a couple living together as man and wife and holding out to the world that the parties are husband and wife. This used to be a widespread practice when the nearest minister was one hundred miles away. With improved transportation and communication, most states have passed laws refusing to recognize common-law marriages, but at least fifteen states still do.

The state has an interest in knowing whether any party has a venereal disease. The law of most states requires a physical examination and blood test of both parties. Other states go beyond this and test for mental disorders, alcoholism, drug addiction, and tuberculosis.

Once the parties take out a marriage license, it is not good forever. Because of the necessity for a medical examination to detect venereal diseases and other diseases sought to be controlled, in most states a marriage license is good for only thirty days. The duration differs in many states; for example, a license is good for only ten days in Louisiana. Some states have a waiting period before a license can be issued, ranging from three to five days.

Of course, a marriage cannot be performed if one of the parties is presently married.

The state has also set rules about the relationship of parties who can marry. Medical tests indicate that persons who are too closely related often have children who are born with hereditary defects. The general rule is that second cousins may marry but no one of closer relationship may.

The marriage ceremony may be solemnized by persons named in the state statutes, usually judges, certain other public officials, ministers, priests, and rabbis.

Property rights are also involved in marriages. When either party acquires property, in most states, the wife acquires dower rights, the life estate to which a married woman is entitled on the death of her husband in lands that her husband owned, and the husband acquires courtesy rights, the life estate to which a married man is entitled on the death of his wife in lands that his wife owned.

It is axiomatic: Marriage is a serious business.

NEGLIGENCE—RIGHTING A WRONG

Nobody is perfect. Even if you do something wrong, you won't be held liable for the result, which could go on and on like a Rube Goldberg project. The law has decided that it is only fair to cut off responsibility in a chain of events at some logical point. Where is the cutoff point?

In many lawsuits, this is the central point to be decided by the court. The law says that to be liable, your wrong must be the "proximate" cause of the injury. What is *proximate cause*? It simply means that you will not be held responsible if the harm you did could not reasonably have been foreseen as a result of the thing you did. If your automobile inspection sticker has expired and someone runs into you without your being at fault otherwise, you would not be responsible because there was no connection between the expired inspection sticker and the collision.

What happens if you have done something wrong but, before

your wrong does any harm, someone else does something wrong that ultimately leads to the accident? Would you be relieved of responsibility? Sometimes. The theory is that your misconduct was not the proximate cause. However, before you can assume that the third party's wrong intervened and relieved you of liability, the court may say that you should have foreseen that such a thing might happen.

OCCUPATIONAL CLAIMS—SORE BACKS AND COMPENSATION

From the beginning of the industrial revolution down to the World War II, if a workman was injured or lost his life on the job, the employer would only be responsible for damages if it could be proven that the employer was negligent, bringing about the injury or death. If proof could not be found, damages could not be awarded even though the workman was totally and permanently injured and his family was thereby forced into poverty. If an injured workman sued his employer, the employer could win the case by showing that the injury was caused by the acts of a fellow workman, that the injured workman was himself negligent and contributed to his own injury, or that the workman knew of the dangers involved in his work and assumed those risks when he took the job. Also, workmen ran the risk of an employer's inability to pay, due to financial instability, if the employee were awarded damages.

Looking at the matter from the employer's viewpoint, many a business was wrecked by a lawsuit brought by an injured employee. The legislatures of the various states took note of the fact that many men would become employers and develop fine businesses but would be apprehensive about hiring employees who might sue them. This whole process caused business and employment to be under-developed.

Laws of most states were changed to introduce a form of insurance to protect the workman and his family, regardless of whether the injury was caused by a fellow workman, the employee had contributed to his own injury, or he had assumed the risk inherent in his employment. Negligence of the employer was no longer important. New laws recognized that the employer must be protected too. The result was a law generally referred to as a Workmen's Compensation Law.

Under this law, an employer with three or more employees is required to carry insurance. If the employer carries the insurance, he is not subject to damage suits by the employee for injuries or death occurring in the employment. Instead, claims are filed with a state agency, and benefits are paid in accordance with a schedule of payments.

All we have said to this point applies to women exactly as it does to men, and injuries to women on the job are equally compensable.

The rates of compensation are fixed by the laws of the individual states. For employee deaths, the decedent's legal beneficiaries are paid weekly, based on a percentage of average wages. If the injury results in partial inability to work, the insurance will pay part of the average weekly wage for a fixed number of weeks. If the workman is so injured that he will not be able to work again, he will be paid a percentage of his average weekly wage for a fixed number of weeks.

Whether a workman or workwoman is partially or totally incapacitated, of course, is a question for determination by the state agency hearing the claim.

Although it has its limitations, the Workmen's Compensation Law protects the workman, his family, and his employer.

PRIVACY—TO BE LET ALONE

Each ten years the federal government conducts a census, which is authorized by the United States Constitution. Most of us don't object to answering the questions that the census poses, but what if you should decide to refuse to answer the questions? Could you do so on the basis that they represent an invasion of your privacy?

This has been answered by the courts, which hold that it is a proper government function and a necessary one to gather reliable statistics that have a bearing on governmental functions, and that intelligent legislation can only be formulated if the government has the facts.

It is probable that people answer the census question because they believe their answers will be kept confidential and that the information will not be used to hurt them. Census answers can't be subpoenaed by parties in a lawsuit and used without the consent of the party giving the answers. However, general statistics can be used, and for the most part, the statistics gathered in the census have been used for the good of all.

RESIDENCE—DOING BUSINESS THERE

Could you open a beauty shop or restaurant in your home or take in typing? Recently, many families have found that their budgets need to be supplemented, and one way is to set up a business in the home.

Neighbors have a different way of looking at it. If the deed to your home contains restrictions—and most of them do—you may find that the restrictions limit your activity to residential use. If you were conducting a business in your home, the court would probably stop you from doing so, even if you continue to reside in your home. The court's attitude is that the basic purpose of maintaining the residential nature of the neighborhood would be violated by your conducting a business there.

What if the thing you are doing in your home is not as apparent as operating a restaurant? Suppose you should elect to teach piano in your home, or take in sewing. The effect of deed restrictions depends on the words of the restrictions, as you might guess, but the minor nature of that activity might and probably would not be stopped by the judge.

It is not a good idea for a person not trained in the law to interpret deed restrictions; before investing in a business to be operated in a home, seek legal advice.

SALES—BUYER BEWARE

For centuries the rule was *caveat emptor*—let the buyer beware. But in recent times, laws have been changed to protect trusting people and prevent action by those who would perpetrate fraud on the public. *Consumer protection* is a term used currently, and many laws have been passed with that aim in mind.

Although consumer protection is a relatively recent concern of government, the Federal Trade Commission, established by Congress in the early 1920s, has been the watchdog of the buying public for many years. Thousands of cases have been brought into the courts by the Federal Trade Commission, ranging from quack medical remedies to false advertising. The Federal Trade Commission has been particularly diligent in its efforts to crack down on false health claims for certain foods and drugs. To be sure, there are things it cannot do, and Congress has laid down rules by which it must conduct its activities. Often the Federal Trade Commission has gone too far, and its activities have been struck down by the courts. More often than not, it has protected one businessman from the fraudulent activities of another, and in recent years it has become the champion of the consumer. Its activities have included banning snake oil to relieve rheumatism, false vitamin claim for artificial orange juice, "French" perfume made in Brooklyn, and so on. The Federal Trade Commission goes to bat for the public if it believes that a wrong has been done.

Caveat emptor was an interesting old idea. Let it rest in peace.

TRAFFIC—RULES OF THE ROAD

In an age when most people drive automobiles, we think everyone is familiar with traffic laws. However, ignorance about use of the public highways is widespread and dangerous.

For example, if at an intersection the traffic control light— which is usually flashing green, amber, and red—should merely be blinking red, it is surprising how many people believe they are entitled to proceed through the intersection without stopping even though the law clearly states that the driver must stop first.

Who has the right-of-way at an intersection where automobiles are approaching and one of them elects to turn left? Is the driver turning left entitled to proceed if he is first in the intersection? No. The driver coming from the opposite direction has the right-of-way even if he is a considerable distance from the crossing, and the driver turning left must yield to him.

What are you to do when you approach an intersection and your light is green but a traffic policeman directs you to stop? In most states you must obey the order of a police officer on the scene rather than the traffic control light.

If an accident occurs, what should you do? The law imposes an obligation to ask whether injuries were suffered and to offer assistance. If the party is injured and one of the automobiles can be driven, the driver should offer to take the injured person to a physician or to a hospital; or if the automobile cannot be driven, he should make an effort to find others who will render assistance to the party injured in the accident.

It should be remembered that statements a person makes at the time of an accident can be used in court. Often, immediately after an accident, the person in a state of anguish misjudges facts thought to be the cause of the accident and makes statements that later prove damaging. Many people conclude that they are at fault and want to confess their error. However, it is wise not to make any statement at all at the time of an accident. Not until all of the facts are known and understood should a person assume responsibility. Especially if the person has liability insurance, he should remember that he owes it to his insurance company to make no statement and to let the company take over the defense of the case.

When a traffic officer investigates an accident, it is his duty to assemble all the facts and preserve them for use by the authorities and the parties involved. In carrying out his duty, the traffic officer will ask each party to make a statement and sign it. It is the better part of wisdom not to make or sign statements at the scene of an accident.

UNEMPLOYMENT COMPENSATION—A HELPING HAND

Unemployment compensation is not a paid vacation. It was designed to bridge the financial gap for those unemployed through no fault of their own. Suppose you were offered a job as a secretary to use a Remington typewriter but refused, saying that you only type with an I.B.M. typewriter. Or suppose you were offered a job as a secretary in a chemical plant but turned it down because you found that you were allergic to the chemicals made there. In which circumstance would you be entitled to unemployment compensation—either or both?

Of course, the rules and regulations with respect to unemployment compensation are not the same in all states. But generally speaking, you can only get unemployment compensation when you refuse a job for which you are not suited. It is highly questionable that you could turn down the secretarial job because your employer didn't offer you the brand of typewriter you preferred—that is pretty unreasonable—but if you turned down the job because you were allergic to the chemicals and this involved a real danger to your health and comfort, this would probably qualify you for unemployment compensation.

If a job required you to stand on your feet for eight hours and by reason of age or infirmity this would be a hardship, your claim would likely be approved, or if the job were located where transportation was not available, this would help your claim.

Of importance, too, are the hours you are required to work and the wages you are offered. If the wages are substantially below those generally offered for work of a similar nature in the place where you live, you would not be required to take the job but could collect unemployment compensation. If you refused a job merely because you wanted to work from eight o'clock to five o'clock and the job required you to work from nine o'clock until six o'clock, this might disqualify your claim.

Each case might be judged on its own facts, but the law seeks to enforce the rule that unemployment compensation is really for people who want to work and not for those who don't.

WOMAN'S AGE—A SECRET

A woman shaves a few years off her age. When is this gentle deception, and when is it fraud?

Before their marriage, Mary told John that she was twenty. After their wedding, he found out she was thirty. Was he defrauded? Does this give him a right to have the marriage set aside? Lengthy court battles have ensued over such issues. Generally, the courts have held that age alone is not the most important thing in a marriage and that although John had not gotten what he bargained for in terms of a younger woman, the courts are hesitant to dissolve marriage on this ground, perhaps because there may be too many cases of it!

If a woman gives an incorrect age on her charge account application, has she committed an offense? Probably not, because her age would not be material to extending credit.

The circumstances would be entirely different, however, in the case of life insurance. Because life insurance is based on risk, which in turn is based on age, an incorrect statement of age inevitably results in a change in the insurance benefits—downward; or if the misstatement of age is material enough in the writing of the policy, the whole policy might be set aside. Insurance companies are very strict about misstatements of age and almost always find out in the end.

Women coyly fib a little about their age and men gallantly look the other way, but the act may not always be frivolous and can have far-reaching consequences.

ENRICHMENT ACTIVITIES

1. **Alimony.**

    Make a list of the factors a judge should take into consideration when fixing the amount of alimony a divorced husband should pay a divorced wife.

2. **Bail.**

    Inquire of the police, sheriff, or constable how you should go about obtaining bail if a member of your family were in jail.

3. **Children.**

    Write a paragraph for, and a paragraph against, the proposition that your neighbor should be liable if his dog bites a child in the neighbor's yard.

4. **Estate Planning.**

    Interview a lawyer or a judge for the unusual results in a case where the decedent left no will.

5. **Food and Drug Laws.**

    Interview a pharmacist for a list of products taken off the market (or restricted to prescriptions) in the last twelve months.

6. **Jury Service.**

    Write your impressions from personal experience (or the experience of someone else) of serving on a jury—the good points and the bad.

7. **Marriage.**

    Ascertain from the town clerk who issues marriage licenses, the minimum age for males, and the minimum age for females to marry, with and without parental consent.

8. **Occupational Claims.**

    Discuss with an insurance agent how workmen's compensation insurance works in your state and how much, and for how long, a workman can receive payments if injured on the job.

9. **Residence.**

    Read a set of deed restrictions (yours or someone else's)

and quote the provision concerning conducting a business in the home.

10. **Traffic.**

Consult the official traffic rule book of your state and quote the rule concerning who has the right of way at an intersection with no stop sign on either street.

glossary

Activity level. The level at which a person burns calories or expends energy to accomplish normal body functions.

Aerobics. Exercise whereby calories are burned by a systematic exercise program including jogging, running, and walking briskly.

Apocrine glands. Producers of perspiration (usually developing an odor) located under the arms.

Articulate. Distinctly uttered.

Articulation. Utterance of articulate sounds, as in pronunciation.

Asymmetrical. Not identical on both sides of a center line.

Athlete's foot. A highly contagious disease characterized by itching, watery blisters, and thick white skin between the toes.

Balance. The state of equilibrium; equal distribution of body weight.

Blush. A red or rosy tint.

Body. A fullness and richness of hair, achieved by back-combing, setting lotions, permanents, and cutting.

Body frame. Size of the body as determined by bone structure; can be small, medium, or large.

Calorie. Heat-producing or energy-producing value in food when oxidized in the body. A unit of the energy supplied by food.

Camouflage. The art of concealing figure faults by proper use of line, color, and texture of fabric; disguise of prominent or unusual features by the use of paint or makeup and hairstyles.

Career. A professional pursuit, such as psychiatry, law, medicine, accounting, or theater, as contrasted with a job; that is, a higher form of human endeavor and pursuit.

Charisma. A magical appeal, possessed in abundance by some individuals.

Chemosurgery. The peeling of skin by the use of chemicals.

Chignon. A coil or knot worn at the crown or nape of the neck (may be a hairpiece).

Cholesterol. A white, fat-soluble substance contained in all animal fats, bile, nervous tissue, blood, gallstones, egg yolk, and so on.

Circulatory. Having to do with the movement of blood through the vessels of the body, induced by the pumping action of the heart.

Color intensity. The brightness or grayness of a color.

Color value. The difference between light and dark tones.

Complementary colors. Colors that fall directly opposite each other on the color wheel.

Compromise. To take the middle road or mid-course instead of an extremity; to pacify and to moderate.

Conditioning. The act of replacing and rebuilding damaged protein structure.

Confidence. Faith and trust in oneself; sureness; positiveness; strength.

Contour. To sketch in outline form; to round off.

Cosmetology. The science of beauty culture practices for skin, complexion, hair, and nails.

Costume. (1) A dress with a jacket or coat that is designed and manufactured together as one ensemble. (2) All the principle pieces of an outfit, including accessories.

Credit. Balance due; the amount a person can obtain from a bank or other business house.

Crown. The upper middle part of the head.

Cuticle. The dead skin that surrounds the edges of the fingernails and toenails. The outer layer of the hair structure.

Cuticle cream. Manicure aid used to correct brittle nails and dry cuticles.

Cuticle oil. Liquid used to soften the skin around the nails.

Dandruff. White or grayish scales formed on the scalp.

Dependent. Relying on another; often used in describing the role of women in traditional marriage; for example, economically dependent.

Depilatory. A cream or liquid substance that removes hair from the body.

Dermabrasion. The removal of outer layers of skin with a small wire brush.

Derrière. The buttocks or rear of the body.

Diaphragm. The partition composed of muscles and sinews that separates the chest from the abdomen.

Diction. Choice of words to express ideas; determining clearness, accuracy, and variety of one's speech.

Eccrine glands. Glands located all over the body that produce odorless perspiration.

Elasticity. Resilience or spring-like quality in hair.

Electrolysis. A method of destroying hair follicles with an electric needle.

Elegant simplicity. The art of dressing tastefully in style and design, free from complexity and becoming the individual and the occasion.

Emerging woman. The phrase used by Jean and Martin Adams in their book, *An Emerging Woman and Her Mate*, to characterize practical or applied women's liberation; a more realistic, practical, and attainable goal for women; evolutionary instead of revolutionary.

Entrepreneur. A self-starter, doer, creator of business and enterprise; an achiever and motivator of others; generally involved with the creation of business to attain economic success.

Eye contact. Looking directly at another person's eyes.

Eye shadow. Color used to color the eyelid and surrounding area.

Fascination. Wonder; amazement; attractiveness.

Feminine. The soft, natural qualities of a woman pertaining to appearance, outlook, attitude, and general conduct.

Feminine passivity. An expression that connotes the nonaggressive role usually associated with women in relationships between the sexes.

Figure analysis. The careful study of the body to determine physical characteristics and to correct figure problems.

Formal. Organized or conditioned behavior.

Frizzy. Having small, tight, fly-away curls.

Goal. An objective one tries to achieve.

Gonorrhea. The most common venereal disease; caused by sexual contact with an infected person; spread by the gonococcus germ, and usually attacking the reproductive system.

Gracefully. Elegantly; with beauty of manner, movement, or speech.

Guest. One who, after accepting the invitation of a host and/or hostess, attends a social gathering.

Gynecologist. A medical doctor who deals with the functions and diseases peculiar to women.

Haircutting. The process of shortening and thinning hair.

Hesitation stance. A gracefully-aligned standing position.

Highlight. The lightest spot or area; to emphasize or focus on.

Horizontal. Situated or arranged on a line parallel to the ground.

Hospitable. Being warm, cordial, friendly, gracious, and generous to guests.

Host. The responsible male at a social gathering.

Hostess. The responsible female at a social gathering.

Hypoallergenic. Containing a less than normal proportion of irritants or allergenic ingredients.

Independent. Able to stand on one's own "two feet;" usually economically self-supporting or self-sufficient.

Isometrics. Exercises whereby one set of muscles is tensed for a period of seconds in opposition to another set of muscles or to a stationary object.

Job. A position with employee status, regular hours, set pay scale, and, in general, predictability, security, routine, order, and following the instructions and policies of other individuals within an organization.

Lease. A contract for the use and possession of real estate for a specified period of time.

Line. The shape of a garment.

Lubricant. A substance that produces an oily film on the surface of the skin and prevents friction.

Magnetism. A unique quality of attraction possessed in larger measure by certain individuals than others.

Maintenance. The upkeep of property.

Manicure. The care of the hands and nails to maintain or improve their appearance.

Mascara. A cosmetic for coloring the eyelashes and eyebrows.

Masculine dominance. A commonly-used expression connoting the male's usually stronger role in occurrences and relationships between the sexes.

Metabolism. The sum of the processes by which a particular substance is handled in the living body. The rate at which a body uses energy.

Moisturizer. A product that adds moisture or water to the skin cells.

Monotoning. Arranging a succession of tints and shades of a single base color.

Monthly statement. Exact record of transactions.

Muscle tone. The condition (firmness) of the body muscles.

Nail buffer. A small, chamois-covered oval block used to smooth nails, create a natural sheen, and stimulate circulation.

Nail matrix. The area at the base of the nail from which the nail itself originates. Only the moon shows; the remainder is underneath the skin in the shape of the nail.

Nape. Back of the neck.

Nasality. The quality of sound uttered through the nose.

Orangewood cuticle stick. A small wooden stick with the end tapered to a forty-five-degree angle.

Pedicure. Procedure for care of the feet and toenails in order to improve their appearance.

Permanent. The changing of straight hair structure into curliness or waviness.

Perseverance. Determination to attain a goal; obstinacy; persistence.

Pitch. The highness or lowness of a sound or tone.

Pivot. A turn-about on one foot.

Plumb line. A cord with a metal bob attached to one end, used to determine verticality.

Poise. A dignified, self-confident manner of self-conduct.

Posture. The body carriage; the position of the limbs.

Primary colors. Blue, yellow, and red; the source of all other colors.

Protein. A complex compound, containing nitrogen, that is a necessary part of animal and plant cells.

Pumice. An abrasive in stone or powder form; used to smooth rough skin on hands or feet and, with a nail buffer, to smooth irregular nail ridges.

Resonance. A vibrating quality of a voice sound; vocal fullness and richness.

Respect. Consideration for another person, expressed in terms of humility, honor, loyalty, and esteem.

Résumé. A summary of personal data, educational background, and business experience.

Rhythm. Movement with uniform or patterned recurrence of a beat or accent, as in walking.

Rinse. To cleanse off soap with repeated applications of water.

Rouge. A cosmetic to color the cheeks or lips red.

Secondary colors. Green, orange, and violet, produced by mixing two primary colors.

Sensitivity. Awareness of other people's feelings; modifying one's conduct according to this awareness.

Service charge. The amount charged for maintaining an account.

Shade. Darker version of a pure color, due to the addition of black; for example, maroon, as compared with clear red.

Shaping. The cutting and molding of hair into a particular style or contour.

Silhouette. The outline or general shape of a garment.

Stance. The position of the body while standing.

Stiff. Overly structured and formal; unrelaxed.

Stride. The length of your step.

Subdue. To reduce the intensity or degree.

Swaybacked. When the back sags to an unusual degree, causing a curvature of the lower part of the spine.

Syphilis. A venereal disease caused by an organism called a spirochete; it can involve every part of the body if not cured; contracted through sexual contact with an infected person.

Texture. The quality and feel of the hair (coarse, medium, or fine); the representation of the structure and minute formation of the skin as distinct from its color.

Tint. Lighter than a natural, pure color (pink as compared to red).

251

Tip. An expression of appreciation for services rendered, normally fifteen percent of the charge.

Tone. A tint or shade of color, especially in makeup and skin pigment.

Torso. The body, excluding the head and limbs.

Total look. The complete appearance of a person, including clothing, accessories, makeup, and hair.

Translucent. Shining or glowing through.

Trim. To balance or even out a present style by lightly cutting the hair.

Trust. Faith in another person or a group, resulting from familiarity, believability, hope, or love.

Venereal disease. A communicable disease, contacted through sexual contact with an infected person.

Vertebrae. The bones or segments composing the spinal column.

Vertical. Upright or plumb.

Virgin hair. Hair that has had no previous bleaching or tinting treatment.

Vitamin. Any of the various organic substances that are essential in minute quantities to the nutrition of the body; they act as regulators to metabolic processes but *do not* provide energy or serve as building units. Vitamins are present in natural foodstuffs and are sometimes produced in the body.

Vocal cords. Two pairs of membranous folds in the larynx, which produce the voice when breath passes between the taut folds of the lower pair.

Wigologist. A person knowledgeable in the care, cutting, and styling of wigs and hairpieces.

Women's Lib. (Women's Liberation Movement) The term used in recent years to describe the women's movement for more freedom in all aspects of life.

index